Pocket Guide to Gastroenterology

Pocket Guide to Gastroenterology

Edited by

David B. Sachar, M.D.
Director, Division of Gastroenterology
The Mount Sinai Hospital
New York, New York

Jerome D. Waye, M.D.
Chief, Gastrointestinal Endoscopy Unit
The Mount Sinai Hospital
New York, New York

Blair S. Lewis, M.D.
Division of Gastroenterology
The Mount Sinai Hospital
New York, New York

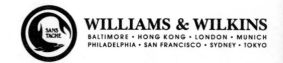

WILLIAMS & WILKINS
BALTIMORE · HONG KONG · LONDON · MUNICH
PHILADELPHIA · SAN FRANCISCO · SYDNEY · TOKYO

Editor: Michael G. Fisher
Associate Editor: Marjorie Kidd Keating
Copy Editor: Miriam L. Kleiger
Design: Dan Pfisterer
Illustration Planning: Wayne Hubbel
Production: Raymond E. Reter

REVISED REPRINT 1991
Copyright © 1989
Williams & Wilkins
428 East Preston Street
Baltimore, Maryland 21202, USA

Accurate indications, adverse reactions, and dosage schedules for drugs are provided in this book, but it is possible that they may change. The reader is urged to review the package information data of the manufaacturers of the medications mentioned.

Printed in the United States of America

Library of Congress Cataloging-in-Publication Data
Formerly titled Gastroenterology for the house officer.
    Includes bibliographies and index.
        1. Gastroenterology—Handbooks, manuals, etc.
2. Digestive organs—Diseases—Handbooks, manuals, etc.
I. Sachar, David B. II. Waye, Jerome D., 1932–   . III. Lewis, Blair S. [DNLM: 1. Digestive System Diseases—physiopathology—handbooks. 2. Digestive System Diseases—therapy—handbooks. WI 39 G257]
RC802.G36   1989   616.3'3   88-28068
ISBN 0-683-07488-1

89 90 91 92 93
1 2 3 4 5 6 7 8 9 10

Preface

If you treat patients with digestive diseases, this book is designed specifically for you. It deals with every common GI problem you are likely to encounter on the wards, in the clinic, or in the emergency room. *Pocket Guide to Gastroenterology* is in fact a guide to the day-to-day practice of gastroenterology, from deciphering "LFTs" to treating constipation, from working up a patient with Crohn's disease to managing a massive GI bleeder.

You will notice, however, that you are not holding in your hands a weighty, comprehensive textbook of gastroenterology. On the contrary, this little volume is a handy pocket reference, written in outline form for quick scanning and for rapid retrieval of key facts. Each problem-oriented section succinctly targets the essentials of history-taking, differential diagnosis, efficient workup and up-to-date therapy. Although we briefly review the basic pathology and pathophysiology of each disorder, our principal focus is always on the practical approach to the patient.

The Mount Sinai Hospital has long been known for its Divisions of Gastroenterology and Liver Disease, but this is the first time we have all written a book together for our favorite audience—our fellow clinicians.

David B. Sachar, M.D.
Jerome D. Waye, M.D.
Blair S. Lewis, M.D.

Contributors

Saul G. Agus, M.D.
Mark L. Chapman, M.D.
Lawrence B. Cohen, M.D.
Nathaniel Cohen, M.D.
Charles D. Gerson, M.D.
Barry Jaffin, M.D.
Henry D. Janowitz, M.D.
Barbara Kapelman, M.D.

Samuel Klein, M.D.
Blair S. Lewis, M.D.
Peter H. Rubin, M.D.
David B. Sachar, M.D.
Robert Shlien, M.D.
Jacob S. Walfish, M.D.
Jerome D. Waye, M.D.

Divisions of Gastroenterology and Liver Disease
The Mount Sinai Hospital
New York, New York

Contents

Chapter 1

Approach to the Patient with Gastrointestinal Symptoms

Henry D. Janowitz, M.D.

I. The Inventory of Complaints: The Cardinal Symptoms

As a House Officer, from the time you begin as a subintern until you finish your training as Senior Resident, you are always facing new patients, daily and nightly, who have gastrointestinal (GI) complaints. Whether in the emergency room (ER), the hospital bed, or the clinic, they do not come labeled as "gastrointestinal" patients, not even in that specialty clinic. If they have been labeled, it is someone else's label. You will need to determine whether their complaints are due to disorders of the gastrointestinal tract and its associated glands (liver and pancreas), or to gastrointestinal reverberations of disorders of other body systems.

Yet the presence of certain cardinal symptoms focuses our attention directly on the gut. Since the GI tract's primary function is the processing of ingested nutrients and fluids in an ordinarily harmonious and unobtrusive fashion, the disruption of this mainly automatic sequence leads to the complaints that bring the patient to us.

Some complaints are plebian, casual, and common: indigestion, or, in more high-toned language, dyspepsia; some are dramatic and life-threatening: bleeding from either end of the tract with vascular collapse; others are more insidious and ominous: loss of appetite and loss of weight. Most insistent and demanding is the presence of pain.

So we may list the cardinal symptoms that make us narrow our focus to the GI tract of our individual patient: *pain* (anywhere along the presumed course of the gut); *bleeding* (grossly obvious to subtly occult); *anorexia, nausea, and weight loss; vomiting, difficulty in swallowing, cramps, diarrhea, constipation* (disturbance of the coordinated movements of the GI tract); *jaundice* (pointing indirectly to the liver, the biliary tree, and the pancreas); and that common but difficult to understand constellation of symptoms, *indigestion, bloating,* and *"gas"* (which probably leads more patients to doctors than any other cause, except perhaps trauma).

II.   Narrative Techniques: The Art of History Taking

Taking the history is the *heart* of the transaction between patient and doctor. It is so important not only because it will lead to the understanding of the patient's illness but also because it is critical for the future productive relationship with the patient: it sets the stage. You will learn more from the patient in the light of the examining room than in the dark of the fluoroscopic room; even in this age of endoscopy, you will learn more from this history than from the light at the end of a long tube.

You must develop your own style of history taking. Observe your mentors, but evolve the style you are comfortable with, adapting it to the urgencies of the situation before you. This means making the patients feel comfortable too. Sit down near them, although there are some limits to informality. The family or friends who accompany the patient or visit at the patient's bedside can be distracting, but they may give you the clinical clue that has been lacking so far.

Unless the immediate situation is life-threatening, let the patients give you their story in their own way. It will be faster that way. Let them read their notes to you, if they have any. Avoid leading questions, at least at the beginning. They can only lead you to your own preconceptions. Remember also the time-honored dictum that if you listen to the patients long enough, they will give you the diagnosis.

In the outpatient setting especially, get a careful inventory of all the medications patients are taking from all the clinics they are attending. You may even have to verify the patients' listing of drugs with their own pharmacists. Drugs may be taken sporadically or intermittently and then forgotten. Although the process is time-consuming, it can be invaluable. This information can be critical, for example, identifying the cause of recurrent pancreatitis.

With individuals not sick enough to be in a hospital bed, take the time to have patients recount an ordinary day's routine of eating and their usual menus. Showing interest in a gastrointestinal patient's nutrition will be rewarded promptly by the patient's confidence. This line of inquiry is most important in deciding to what extent malnutrition and malabsorption are each contributing to the patient's weight loss.

In this context, getting a patient's weight in a hospital may often be difficult, but it provides extremely useful and sometimes critical information.

III. The Heart of the Physical Examination: A Scanning Technique

If the history has fixed your attention on the possible role of the GI tract, then your physical examination will lead you to focus more directly on certain areas of the patient. You will not neglect other aspects, but you are more likely to pick up some clue if you know what you are looking for.

Examine the *sclera* and *skin* by daylight, near a window if need be. It is embarrassing to miss jaundice by yellow electric light.

In the skin, the lesions of erythema nodosum and pyoderma gangrenosum of inflammatory bowel disease present no problem of recognition. The early thickening of the skin of the face or hands in *scleroderma* may be most subtle. The mottled skin of *livido reticulosis* in acute pancreatitis is a useful finding, as is the ecchymosis of the flank or abdominal wall in that disorder. Any abdominal wall scar raises the possibility of a mechanical obstruction due to adhesions or bands.

Clubbing of the fingertips and curvature of the nails occur in small bowel disease and in cirrhosis, as well as in pulmonary and congestive heart disease, but always inquire about the family history of clubbing so as not to be led astray. The nails may help in chronic liver disease. The presence of psoriasis of skin and nails can be associated with Crohn's disease.

In all syndromes that sound functional, look carefully for physical signs of Graves' disease.

When you look at the tongue for its papillation, you should

then be looking at the mouth for the aphthous ulcers of Crohn's disease as well as for the rare thickening of lips and gums in that disease.

Listen to the abdomen before palpating it. Most midline noises are meaningless. The left upper quadrant bruit caused by turbulence in the splenic vessels is classic for cancer of the pancreas. Listening in the flank, you may discover the bruit of renal vascular abnormalities.

Elicit a succussion splash if you can, but be sure that the patient has not eaten recently. A splash in the left upper quadrant is characteristic of gastric outlet obstruction, but other splashes can be heard throughout the abdomen in cases of small bowel obstruction of any cause. Do not forget to examine the umbilicus for metastatic cancer and herniation. The presence of an inguinal hernia may point to a cause for intermittent partial small bowel obstruction or to the presence of a cancer of the colon.

Gastroenterologists are permitted to listen above the diaphragm. Aortic stenosis of any variety may be present and points to arteriovenous malformation along the entire GI tract in bleeding of unknown origin. Mitral valve prolapse has been associated with some functional bowel syndromes, especially colonic inertia.

For right upper quadrant pain simulating biliary tract disease or left upper quadrant diseases simulating the "splenic flexure" syndrome, use the "hooking" maneuver to elicit pain from a slipped 10th or 11th rib.

The dilated veins of portal hypertension, the cluster around the umbilicus (the caput medusae), gross ascites, and the enlarged liver and/or spleen of cirrhosis are obvious findings, but the detection of small amounts of fluid in the peritoneum is difficult. Distinguishing an abdomen distended by peritoneal fluid from one distended by fluid- or air-filled bowel is not easy.

Learn to do a careful rectal examination, and go to the rectal clinic if necessary to learn how. Using a head mirror with reflected light leaves both hands free to look for fissures and hemorrhoids. These are more common causes of rectal pain and bleeding than cancer.

IV. Formulating the Problems

Having finished your history taking and the physical examination of the patient, you should summarize in capsule form your findings and the possible diagnoses that have occurred to you during the course of the transaction so far. It is important to do this immediately because you will never have another opportunity to do so with your impressions as fresh as they are now.

First, formulate the problem or problems the patient presents. Are you facing:

A swallowing problem;
Gastrointestinal bleeding;
A diarrhea problem;
Intraabdominal inflammation;
Intestinal pain due to reflux mechanism;
Complete or incomplete intestinal obstruction;
Obstipation and constipation;
Anorexia with weight loss;
Nausea and vomiting;
Intraabdominal infection or abscess;
Malnutrition; or
Malabsorption?

Then list your possible diagnoses in the order you consider most probable. I believe most errors in diagnosis are errors of omission. We do not spread our nets wide enough.

V. Priorities: Diagnostic and Therapeutic

While outlining your plan of diagnostic investigation, parallel it with your possible plan for treatment. There are important diagnostic lessons to be learned from the patient's response to therapy, and this may earn the patient's confidence. Recognize the patient not as a puzzle but as someone who is hurting.

Do something for the patient even in the first interview. This is especially important for the patient in the hospital; do something for him or her every day, even if it is only ordering a hot water bottle or having a chat. Remember, the hospital patient awaits your coming all day.

VI. Current Diagnostic Technology

In the presence of ever-multiplying methods for investigating the disorders of the GI tract, it is helpful to divide these methods into several categories. Some are the *ABCs* and some are the *XYZs*. The *ABCs* include the blood count, with the smear, to determine the presence of anemia of blood loss or chronic inflammation, the leukocytosis of acute suppuration; and the digital rectal exam, which should always include the effort to obtain stool for testing for occult blood. I perform routine proctoscopy (and/or sigmoidoscopy) if this can be arranged at the first clinical examination. Thyroid function studies are in order.

The *XYZs* of technology include the invasive or extensive procedures such as endoscopy, endoscopic retrograde cholangiopancreatography (ERCP), computed tomography (CT) scanning, nuclear magnetic resonance (NMR) imaging, and percutaneous transhepatic catheterization. Classical radiography with barium, abdominal ultrasonography, and radionuclide scanning are intermediates.

I have found also that any form of discussion of the diagnostic techniques is helpful not only for the physician but also for the patient. They easily grasp the differences between methods that evaluate structure (the "parts" of the human machine) and those that evaluate *function* (how the "parts" are working).

The *structural* techniques range from x-rays and sonography, through endoscopy, to biopsy. The easily available *functional* ones include manometric measurement of pressure at either end of the GI tract (esophagus and rectum); marker tests of transit time; absorption studies; D-xylose, vitamin B_{12}, fecal fats, stool electrolytes; biliary scanning; serum assays (gastrin, vasoactive intestinal peptide (VIP), parathyroid hormone (PTH), and serotonin). Structural and functional studies may parallel each other, but they need care in their scheduling to prevent conflicts and delays. The barium studies so easily available can hold up endoscopy, sonography, and CT scanning, as well as the careful examination of the stool for parasites and pathogens.

VII. Some Obiter Dicta

There are few periodic pains of gastrointestinal origin that awaken patients regularly from sleep. Peptic ulcerations of stomach and duodenum, as well as cancer of the pancreas, are the commonest. The irritable bowel rarely awakens the patient in the middle of the night. *Proctalgia fugax,* a fleeting, lightning-like intense rectal spasm, can also occur in the middle of the night; it resembles nocturnal leg cramps.

The onset of the acute pain of biliary colic or pancreatitis is to be related to the time of eating the offending meal or the taking of excessive alcohol. Biliary colic pains rarely occur early in the morning.

Nausea, especially nausea without vomiting, is one of the most difficult symptoms to manage and treat. Nausea that has an organic basis rises most often from the duodenum via vagal afferents: remember that of the 40,000 vagal fibers, 36,000–38,000 are afferents to the brain stem. Although giardiasis causes nausea, and the organism does live in the duodenum, the infection is usually accompanied by small bowel symptoms of diarrhea and cramps.

The classical location of a pain is classic because the pain most often does occur in the expected location, but the atypical does exist: Sigmoid diverticulitis pain may occur in the right lower quadrant and mimic appendicitis. A slow leak from a duodenal ulcer may track down to the right lower quadrant and simulate appendicitis. Recurrent appendicitis secondary to a fecalith is rare but does occur.

Distinguish *osmotic* from *secretory* diarrhea. *Osmotic* diarrhea occurs when the patient is fed by mouth; it rarely occurs during the night. The *secretory* form continues even when the patient receives calories and fluid only by vein. The secretory form is rare, and is usually due to circulatory hormone factors (VIP, catecholamines, etc.). Laxative abuse and surreptitious use of diuretics are more common. Add some sodium hydroxide to the stool to elicit the pink color of phenolphthalein present in many laxatives.

Despite the everpresent possibility of factitious (man- or woman-made) disease, believe the patient, particularly when she or he has discovered a mass.

In sorting out the diarrheal diseases, especially in the absence of gross bleeding, smears of the stools for leukocytes are invaluable in recognizing bowel inflammation.

In gastrointestinal bleeding of unknown origin, when barium contrast films and extensive endoscopy have failed to pinpoint the source, labeled red cell scans are useful. Angiography alone has often not helped unless the red cell scans are positive.

Chapter 2

Disorders of the Esophagus

Barry Jaffin, M.D.

I. Introduction

The esophagus, once thought of as a long, static cylindrical tube connecting the mouth to the stomach, has over the last 5 to 10 years taken on an importance of its own. This is attributable to newer technologies available for evaluating patients with atypical chest pain. In addition, the large number of immunocompromised patients who present with esophageal symptoms has caused attention to be focused on this organ.

II. Dysphagia

A. Definition

Dysphagia is the subjective sensation of impairment in the transport of a bolus of food into the esophagus. The conditions that result in dysphagia can be subdivided into: diseases that anatomically affect the oropharynx (myasthenia gravis, polymyositis, amyotrophic lateral sclerosis (ALS), Parkinson's disease, and cranial nerve palsies); and disorders that affect the thoracic esophagus. The latter group can be subdivided into disorders causing: (*a*) mechanical dysfunction: carcinoma, webs, strictures, or extraluminal obstruction by tumor or lymph nodes; (*b*) motor dysfunction: motility disturbances such as achalasia, scleroderma, esophageal spasm, nutcracker esophagus, diabetic neuropathy, and amyloidosis; and (*c*) mucosal dysfunction: disorders such as esophagitis (acid reflux), infectious diseases (e.g., those due to cytomegalovirus (CMV), herpes, and Candida), and inflammatory diseases (e.g., Crohn's disease).

B. Differential Diagnosis

Dysphagia for solid foods generally implies mechanical obstruction due to mucosal webs (if nonprogressive) or carcinoma (if progressive). Strictures due to acid reflux disease can be progressive and can mimic symptoms of carcinoma, including weight loss.

C. Diagnostic Tests

A menu of tests is available to help identify the cause of dysphagia:

1. Cineesophagram. Useful in evaluating patients with cervical dysphagia, since the radiologist is able to film the sequence of pharyngeal contraction and upper esophageal sphincter relaxation.

2. Endoscopy. This procedure enables the gastroenterologist to diagnose esophageal lesions such as carcinoma, strictures, webs, or esophagitis.

3. Esophageal Motility. This test may be of help in determining the coordination of pharyngeal contraction and upper sphincter relaxation. It will give direct measurements of the contraction wave (amplitude and duration) and sphincter pressure.

III. **Chest Pain**

A. Overview

Nearly 30% of the 750,000 cardiac catheterizations performed annually in the United States reveal no significant coronary artery disease. This implies a large number of patients whose pain may be of esophageal origin. Symptoms in these patients can include heartburn, dysphagia (difficulty in swallowing), odynophagia (painful swallowing), and regurgitation. Gastroesophageal reflux disease (GERD) and esophageal motor disorders account for most esophageal chest pain syndromes.

B. Gastroesophageal Reflux Disease (GERD)—Heartburn

1. Pathophysiologic factors may include:

   a. Decreased amplitude of the lower esophageal sphincter (fats, chocolates, carminatives, xanthines, calcium channel blockers, anticholinergics, prostaglandins (E_2)).
   b. Impaired esophageal acid clearance.
   c. Decreased salivation.
   d. Decreased amplitude of esophageal contraction.
   e. Increased sensitivity of receptors on the esophageal mucosa (e.g., to citrus fruits).
2. Tests to evaluate GERD include:
   a. Barium Esophagram/Fluoroscopy. Usually the first test performed to exclude organic lesions of the esophagus and stomach. The patient should be examined in the supine and upright positions.
   b. Endoscopy. Very helpful in excluding organic lesions of the upper gastrointestinal (GI) tract. Excellent for evaluating the gastroesophageal (GE) junction and ruling out Barrett's esophagus (replacement of the squamous mucosa with columnar epithelium). Barrett's epithelium may give rise to adenocarcinoma.
   c. Esophageal Motility. Helpful in detecting dysfunction of the body of the esophagus. Patients with reflux usually have resting pressures of the lower sphincter less than 12 mm Hg compared to a gastric baseline of zero.
   d. Acid Perfusion Test (Bernstein). A solution of 0.1 M hydrochloric acid is dripped into the distal esophagus at a rate of 8 cc/minute. A positive test reproduces the patient's pain complex. Normal saline is used as a placebo.
   e. Esophageal pH Measurements (24 Hours). This test is used to document the number and frequency of reflux episodes (usually defined as pH less than 4.0). Episodes can be correlated to patient's syndrome. This test is becoming the gold standard for defining acid reflux disease.
   f. Gastroesophageal Scintigraphy. A noninvasive test that evaluates esophageal emptying using radioisotopes.
3. Treatment of GERD.
   a. Dietary adjustment is the first step. It is important to avoid foods that lower the lower esophageal sphincter

pressure (coffee, chocolates, alcohol, tomatoes, pepper-mints, oils). Mechanical measures are also important: weight loss, avoidance of tight-fitting garments, and elevation of the head of the bed (not just adding pillows).

b. The next step includes the use of antacids (after meals or when symptomatic), H-2 blockers (cimetidine, ranitidine, famotidine), or Carafate (generic name: sucralfate). The latter are usually given after dinner or prior to bedtime.

c. If the above measures are not helpful, the addition of a prokinetic agent such as metoclopramide (a dopamine antagonist) or bethanechol (a cholinergic agonist) is useful. One must watch for side effects such as tardive dyskinesia for the former, or parasympathetic effects for the latter. Domperidone is a medication similar to metoclopramide, but it does not cross the blood-brain barrier, and it thus avoids many of the side effects of metoclopramide. It is already used in many countries (under the trade name Motilium), and it is expected to become available in the United States soon. On the horizon is a new medication, cisapride, which appears to have stronger prokinetic action than metoclopramide without either antidopaminergic or cholinergic effects.

d. Finally, if patients are debilitated by severe esophagitis, aspiration pneumonia, or disabling symptoms, then antireflux surgery (i.e., Nissen fundoplication) should be considered.

C. Esophageal Motility Disorders
Esophageal motility disorders can cause chest pain and should be looked for if gastroesophageal reflux disease is not present. The following motor disorders can cause chest pain:

1. Achalasia. Defined manometrically as aperistalsis of the esophageal body (required for diagnosis), incomplete relaxation of the lower sphincter to swallows, and elevated lower sphincter pressure (usually greater than 40 mm Hg). This pattern is seen in fewer than 10% of patients presenting with esophageal chest pain.

a. Symptoms. Dysphagia, regurgitation, chest pain.
b. Pathology. Loss of Auerbach's plexus in the body of the

esophagus and lower esophageal sphincter area.
   c. X-ray Findings. Absence of esophageal peristalsis, dilated esophagus with a smoothly tapered "bird beak" appearance, loss of gastric air fluid level on chest x-ray.
2. Diffuse Esophageal Spasm. Manometrically defined as simultaneous contractions (greater than 10% of swallows) and intermittent normal peristalsis. Simultaneous contractions are esophageal contractions that occur all at once up and down the length of the esophagus; they are independent of pharyngeal contractions and are nonperistaltic. Normal peristalsis should be seen intermittently in order to make the diagnosis of diffuse esophageal spasm. Diagnosis is based on the absence of organic lesions. This pattern is seen in 10 to 15% of patients with noncardiac chest pain. Symptoms may be precipitated by cold fluids and emotional stress.
3. Nutcracker Esophagus. Manometrically defined as normal peristalsis with a mean amplitude of distal esophageal contractions greater than 180 mm Hg (greater than two standard deviations above mean). Increased duration of contraction may be seen (greater than 6 months). This pattern is most commonly seen in patients with noncardiac chest pain. The use of edrophonium chloride (Tensilon test) will increase the amplitude and duration of esophageal contraction in both normal patients and patients with esophageal motility disorders. A positive test will simulate the patient's chest pain complex independently of the motility tracing. Normal saline should be used as a placebo.
4. Nonspecific Esophageal Motility Disorder (NEMD). Any combination of the following manometric parameters: intermittent normal peristalsis, simultaneous contractions (greater than 10%), nontransmitted contractions (greater than 10% of swallows), triple peaked contractions, or a mean distal esophageal amplitude less than 30 mm Hg. This pattern is commonly seen in patients with noncardiac chest pain, and in patients with dysphagia.
5. Secondary Motor Disorders. Scleroderma is a disease of unknown etiology which involves the esophagus. Manifestations include dysphagia for liquids and solids. Involvement is characterized by a reduction of the lower esophag-

eal sphincter pressure and a decrease in the amplitude of esophageal contraction. This leads to distal esophagitis and stricture formation. H-2 blockers should be given to prevent esophagitis.

6. Treatment of Esophageal Motility Disorders. A trial of the following medications is in order. Nitroglycerin (0.4 mg sublingually 30 minutes prior to meals and at night), or isorbide dinitrate (10–30 mg orally 30 minutes prior to meals) can be tried in any esophageal motility disorder that has an increased amplitude of contraction, since these medications have been shown to decrease the amplitude of esophageal contraction. Calcium channel blockers such as nifedipine (10–30 mg sublingually 30 minutes prior to meals and at bedtime) or diltiazem (60–90 mg orally 30 minutes prior to meals) are appropriate. Smooth muscle relaxants, e.g., hydralazine, are rarely used. Dilatation using bougienage with a Maloney dilator greater than 50 French, or pneumatic dilatation, can be used in patients with achalasia or in patients with a hypertensive lower esophageal sphincter pressure.

IV. Odynophagia

Odynophagia is defined as painful swallowing; it may be caused by any inflammatory condition of the esophagus. Infectious disorders are now the most common etiologies among immunocompromised patients. Reflux esophagitis is seen frequently in nonimmunocompromised patients.

A. Candidiasis
  1. Pathogenesis. Predisposing factors include malignancy, diabetes, antibiotics, steroids, and immunocompromised states.
  2. Diagnosis. Diagnosis of esophagitis can be made on barium swallow, although a specific diagnosis of candidiasis is difficult. The mucosal pattern may reveal ulcerations. Endoscopy will reveal whitish plaques with normal mucosal pattern between the plaques. Direct smears (brush) are more sensitive than biopsy. Silver methenamine stain brings out yeast forms. Serum agglutinins are not helpful.
  3. Treatment. Therapy consists of a trial of Nystatin 250,000 units suspension in water or mixed in methyl cellulose every

2 hours. Clotrimazole troches can be given every 2 hours. Ketoconazole 200 mg per day or low-dose amphotericin B given intravenously can be used if the above medications do not ameliorate the patient's symptoms.

B. Herpetic Esophagitis
   1. Pathogenesis. Predisposing factors include lymphoma, leukemia, or any immunocompromised state.
   2. Diagnosis. Diagnosis usually rests on endoscopy. Separate ulcers or shallow plaques are seen. Biopsy reveals inclusion bodies within epithelial cells. Multinucleated giant cells should be seen.
   3. Treatment. Therapy consists of symptomatic treatment using viscous Xylocaine. Experimental drugs (D.N.P.G.) have been used in CMV esophagitis with some success.

V. Esophageal Bleeding

Hematemesis is the act of vomiting blood. The specific source of blood loss should be determined. Bleeding can arise from the oropharynx or nasal passages and should not be overlooked. Bleeding from the esophagus may be due to inflammatory, neoplastic, or vascular causes.

A. Bleeding Esophageal Varices
   1. Pathogenesis. Cirrhosis of the liver causes increased portal pressure, which is transmitted to the preexisting collateral channels to dilate the esophageal veins. Alcohol is the most common etiologic agent causing cirrhosis in the United States.
   2. Clinical Presentation. Although varices may be asymptomatic, life-threatening bleeding may occur; this appears to be related to the size of the varix. There is usually a concurrent coagulopathy due to underlying liver disease and a thrombocytopenia due to hypersplenism.
   3. Treatment. Replacement of blood volume with packed red blood cells (RBCs) and hydration is most important. Correction of the coagulopathy with fresh frozen plasma may be helpful. Endoscopic modalities include sclerotherapy with injection of a sclerosing agent. Sengstaken-Blakemore tube has been used in the past with success. Intravenous vasopressin has shown mixed results, yet it is used frequently.

B. Mallory-Weiss Tear (MWT)
  1. Pathogenesis. This mucosal tear is produced by transmural pressure gradients usually associated with retching and vomiting. Associated conditions include the presence of a hiatus hernia.
  2. Clinical Presentation. Eighty percent of MWTs will occur along the lesser curve of the stomach. Ten percent will involve the esophagus. Males predominate. Alcohol is common.
  3. Treatment. Most Mallory-Weiss tears will heal spontaneously. Ten percent may require therapeutic endoscopic measures, i.e., heater probe, monopolar coagulation.

VI. **Miscellaneous Esophageal Disorders**

  A. Esophageal Web
    1. Pathogenesis. An esophageal web is a mucosal structure located anywhere along the esophagus. Reflux esophagitis may play a role in the development of a web.
    2. Clinical Presentation. Intermittent dysphagia, non-progressive in nature. If the web is located in the cervical esophagus and is associated with iron deficiency, the condition may be referred to as the Plummer-Vinson syndrome. This syndrome is associated with achlorhydria, glossitis, and stomatitis. If the ring (web) is located in the distal esophagus, the condition may be called the steak house syndrome.
    3. Treatment. Bougienage with Maloney dilators has been the mainstay in therapy. Newer dilators, which can be passed through an endoscope (TTS), are now in use.
  B. Zenker's Diverticulum
    1. Pathogenesis. This hypopharyngeal diverticulum is thought to be associated with a dysfunctioning upper esophageal sphincter. The precise mechanism is unknown.
    2. Clinical Presentation. Patients usually present with cervical dysphagia, halitosis, or aspiration pneumonia. This type of diverticulum is usually found in men over 50 years of age. The diagnosis may be made by barium swallow.
    3. Treatment. Usually none. If disabling aspiration pneumonia keeps recurring, surgery can be considered.
  C. Caustic Ingestions

1. Clinical Presentation. Ingestion of alkali or acid compounds results in injury to the esophagus or stomach. Odynophagia is the most common symptom, while laryngeal stridor is uncommon. There may be a poor correlation of symptoms and extent of injury.
2. Treatment. All patients should be kept NPO and should be given intravenous hydration. Endoscopy should be performed unless there is evidence of a perforation or extensive necrosis. Steroids and antibiotics have been empirically used to prevent fibrosis and infection, although no controlled trials are available to support their role.

D. Acute Esophageal Obstruction
1. Clinical Presentation. Patients usually have prior symptoms of heartburn, dysphagia, or odynophagia suggesting underlying esophageal pathology.
2. Treatment. Pharmacologic agents (glucagon 1 mg intravenously or NTG 0.6 mg sublingually) relaxes the lower esophageal sphincter and may allow passage of the bolus of food. Endoscopy can be diagnostic (carcinoma/stricture), and therapeutic, by allowing either extraction of the foreign body, or else the crushing and then pushing of the foreign body into the stomach, depending on the type of foreign body and the etiology of the obstruction. Papain or meat tenderizers should be avoided. Avoid maneuvers that increase the risk of aspiration, e.g., barium swallow.

VII. Premalignant Disorders of the Esophagus

A. Lye Ingestion
Increased incidence of squamous cell carcinoma usually within 20–25 years following ingestion. There is controversy concerning whether surveillance should begin after 20 years.
B. Achalasia
Increased risk of squamous cell carcinoma of the esophagus. It is unclear whether or not treatment for achalasia alters the incidence of carcinoma.
C. Barrett's Esophagus
Barrett's esophagus is defined as epithelial metaplasia in which specialized columnar epithelium is replaced by stratified squamous epithelium. This metaplasia may occur in up to 10% of patients with chronic reflux. The lifetime risk of developing

adenocarcinoma is reported to range from 3 to 5%. Medical or surgical antireflux therapy does not appear to reduce the risk of carcinoma. Surveillance is controversial; consider endoscopic biopsy every 1–2 years.

D. Tylosis

A rare condition, which is manifested as thickened skin on the hands and feet and is associated with an increased risk of esophageal carcinoma.

E. Plummer-Vinson Syndrome

A condition that is associated with an increased incidence of esophageal carcinoma.

SUGGESTED READINGS

Castell DO, Richter JE, Dalton CB: *Esophageal Motility Testing.* New York, Elsevier, 1987.

Levine J: *Decision Making in Gastroenterology.* Saint Louis, CV Mosby, 1985.

Chapter 3

Acute Gastrointestinal Bleeding

Lawrence B. Cohen, M.D.
Blair S. Lewis, M.D.

As a house officer in the emergency room or at the beside, you will often be involved in the care of patients with gastrointestinal (GI) hemorrhage. You'll no doubt remember the first time you were called to evaluate a patient with hematemesis or massive hematochezia. It is important in the face of such a dire emergency to keep your wits about you and think of the basic things that need to be done to stabilize, diagnose, and treat the patient.

APPROACH TO THE PATIENT

I. **Initial Assessment and Resuscitation**

    A. Hemodynamic Status

        1. Vital Signs. The first step in the management of an acutely ill patient is to ensure that the vital organs of the body (heart, lungs, brain, and kidneys) are receiving adequate blood flow. This assessment is accomplished by evaluating the vital signs.

            a. Pulse and blood pressure should be taken in the supine and upright positions. A fall in the blood pressure of more than 10 mm Hg or a rise of more than 20 beats/minute in

the pulse rate between the supine and standing positions is indicative of an acute loss of at least 20% of the intravascular blood volume.
   b. Hypovolemic shock associated with hypotension, tachycardia, and impaired mental state indicates an acute blood loss of 40% or more of the blood volume.
   c. Respiratory distress is unusual during GI hemorrhage and often signals an aspiration pneumonia.
2. Cutaneous signs of peripheral vasoconstriction include pallor, diaphoresis, and livido reticulosis.
3. Level of consciousness may be altered due to reduced cerebral blood flow.
4. Urine Output. A urine output of less than 30 ml/hour indicates inadequate perfusion of the kidneys.
B. Resuscitative Measures
   1. Intravenous Access.
      a. The first order of business is hemodynamic resuscitation. A large-bore intravenous catheter should be inserted immediately upon arrival of the patient in the emergency room.
      b. When the catheter is inserted, blood should be obtained for a hematocrit, and specimens sent to the laboratory for additional tests (see below).
      c. Peripheral access is preferable to a central venous line since flow is slower across the longer and narrower central venous pressure (CVP) catheter. It is rarely necessary to monitor CVP or pulmonary artery pressures in patients with bleeding. An exception to this is the elderly patient with reduced cardiac reserve and congestive heart failure.
   2. Volume.
      a. Intravenous fluids should be rapidly administered using normal saline, particularly if the patient is hypotensive.
      b. The administration of large volumes of crystalloid may lead to the formation or worsening of ascites in patients with liver disease and should, therefore, be limited in such patients.
   3. Blood Products.
      a. Packed Red Blood Cells (PRBC). In most cases of GI hem-

orrhage, the blood product of choice for transfusion is PRBC. When a patient is hypotensive from blood loss, transfusion should be performed as soon as cross-matched blood is available. In an emergency situation, it may be necessary to transfuse type-specific blood (type O). In the absence of active blood loss, the hematocrit should rise by 3 points for each unit of transfused blood. One unit of fresh frozen plasma and 1 gram of calcium gluconate should be administered after every 4 units of PRBC.

    b. Fresh Frozen Plasma. In general, this should only be given to patients with active bleeding and a coagulopathy.

    c. Platelets. A platelet transfusion is indicated for the bleeding patient whose platelet count is less than 20,000.

  4. Pressor Agents. Pressors are rarely helpful in patients whose primary problem is intravascular blood loss.

  5. Airway Protection. The patient with a reduced level of consciousness and repeated episodes of vomiting may require intubation to protect the airway and prevent aspiration of gastric contents.

  6. Oxygen. Oxygen should be administered to patients with hypotension via nasal cannula at 5–10 L/minute.

C. Monitoring of Patient (Fig. 3.1)

All patients with GI bleeding should be followed with a detailed flow sheet that charts their course and provides an ongoing assessment of their condition. Patients with active GI bleeding should be admitted to an intensive care unit to facilitate close supervision.

II. Taking the History

  A. History of Present Illness

    1. Painful versus painless bleeding.

      a. Painful.

        i. Upper tract: peptic ulcer disease, esophagitis, tumors.

        ii. Lower tract: colitis, ischemia.

      b. Painless.

        i. Upper tract: varices, angiodysplasia.

        ii. Lower tract: diverticulosis, angiodysplasia, neoplasm, hemorrhoids.

Date											
Time											
Vital Signs											
BP											
P											
Urine Output (ml/hr)											
Mental Status											
CBC											
Hgb											
Hct											
Plt											
PT											
Electrolytes											
K											
BUN											
Cr											
Ca											
Blood Products											
PC											
FFP											
Plt											
IV											
Type											
Rate (ml/hr)											
Meds											

Figure 3.1.   Flow sheet for patients with GI bleeding.

2. Quantitate the volume and duration of blood loss. An estimate should be made of the total amount of blood loss which has occurred. This estimate can be deduced from the frequency, duration, and volume of bleeding. Patients often overestimate the amount of blood loss which has taken place.

B. History of Previous GI Bleeding

A history of prior GI hemorrhage may suggest the cause of the present bleeding episode. However, it is important to recognize that patients may bleed from unrelated sites on different occasions. For example, patients with known esophageal varices and an acute hemorrhage will be bleeding from a nonvariceal cause at least 20% of the time.

C. Pertinent Medical History

Other medical disorders may predispose to GI hemorrhage:

Chronic renal failure
Diabetes mellitus
Chronic obstructive lung disease
Peripheral vascular disease
Chronic liver disease
Osler-Weber-Rendu syndrome
Valvular heart disease

D. History of Bleeding Diathesis

A history of known bleeding disorders should always be sought. Easy bruisability or protracted bleeding after minor surgical procedures or dental extractions may indicate the presence of a bleeding diathesis.

E. Medications, Toxins, and Alcohol

Ingested substances that may be associated with GI hemorrhage can be divided into several categories:

1. Medications causing GI ulceration.
   a. Nonsteroidal anti-inflammatory drugs (including aspirin).
   b. Methotrexate.
2. Medications that promote bleeding.
   a. Antiplatelet drugs.
   b. Anticoagulants.
3. Alcohol, both by direct effect on the GI mucosa and indirectly by producing liver injury, portal hypertension, and impaired coagulation.

F. Family Medical History

GI hemorrhage may be the first manifestation of a heritable bleeding dyscrasia or GI disease for which there is a positive family history.

G. Allergies

A history of allergy to medications should be obtained prior to the administration of any pharmacologic agents.

III. Physical Examination

A. Vital Signs (see above)

B. Mental Status

In a patient with GI bleeding, the following causes of altered sensorium should initially be considered:

1. Hypotension.
2. Intoxication due to alcohol or other agents.
3. Hepatic encephalopathy.
4. Renal insufficiency.
5. Hyper- or hypoglycemia.
6. Cerebrovascular accident or subdural hematoma.

C. Stigmata of Chronic Liver Disease

Jaundice, cutaneous angiomata, palmar erythema, gynecomastia, enlargement of the parotid glands, and testicular atrophy are findings suggestive of chronic liver disease. Esophageal varices are likely to be present when other signs of portal hypertension, such as splenomegaly, ascites, and caput medusae, are present.

D. Integument

Multiple ecchymoses, petechiae, or telangiectasia may indicate the presence of a disorder of hemostasis. There are also a number of systemic diseases that are associated both with GI bleeding and skin lesions.

E. Nose and Throat

Careful examination of the nasopharynx and throat should be performed, since profuse bleeding from these areas may result in melena or hematemesis. Trauma to the nasal turbinates during passage of a nasogastric tube may produce considerable bleeding.

F. Abdomen

Hepatosplenomegaly, prior surgical scars, and signs of ascites are all important findings. Localized abdominal tenderness

may help in the assessment of a bleeding patient.
- G. Lymphatics
  The presence of either regional or generalized adenopathy may suggest the presence of an underlying systemic disease.
- H. Rectal Examination
  The color of the stool should be noted and the presence of a rectal mass ruled out.

IV. Laboratory Studies

- A. Complete Blood Count
  1. The hemoglobin and hematocrit may be normal during an acute hemorrhage, since it can take up to 6 hours for equilibration of the intravascular space.
  2. Thrombocytosis may occur with acute bleeding. A low platelet count in a patient with intestinal bleeding may be due to hypersplenism, a disorder of platelet consumption (e.g., disseminated intravascular coagulation), or a primary thrombocytopenic condition.
- B. Prothrombin Time (PT) and Partial Thromboplastin Time (PTT)
  An assessment of the coagulation status should include a prothrombin time and partial thromboplastin time.
  1. Prolongation of the PT may result from use of dicumarol, liver disease, disorders of fat malabsorption, and prolonged administration of antibiotics.
  2. Abnormalities of the PTT are usually the consequence of either congenital or acquired disorders of hemostasis such as factor VIII deficiency, von Willebrand's disease, and disseminated intravascular coagulation.
  3. Additional parameters of clotting such as the bleeding time and thrombin time may be necessary when a bleeding diathesis is suspected.
- C. Serum Electrolytes
  The electrolytes should be followed closely when a patient is receiving large amounts of fluid and blood or a nasogastric tube is used for continuous suctioning. Lactic acidosis may result from prolonged hypotension or ischemia, while hypochloremic alkalosis may occur during prolonged nasogastric aspiration.
- D. Glucose and Calcium

Hypoglycemia may develop in patients with chronic liver disease, or hyperglycemia may develop in the chemical diabetic following administration of large volumes of dextrose-containing fluids. Hypocalcemia can arise during large-volume blood transfusions.

E. Blood Urea Nitrogen (BUN) and Creatinine

A disproportionate rise in BUN compared with creatinine (ratio greater than 20:1) suggests that the site of bleeding is within the upper GI tract. Renal failure is often associated with GI bleeding.

F. Peripheral Blood Smear

The blood smear may provide important information regarding the chronicity of the blood loss (microcytic anemia) or the presence of an underlying hematologic or liver disorder.

G. Liver Chemistries

A marked elevation of the serum transaminases is found following a period of hypoperfusion of the liver (shock liver). Abnormal liver chemistries may suggest the presence of underlying liver disease.

H. Electrocardiogram

An electrocardiogram should be performed prior to any invasive diagnostic tests to exclude the presence of coronary ischemia due to hypotension.

V. Diagnostic Procedures in Acute Gastrointestinal Bleeding

A. Initial Evaluation

In order to achieve prompt and effective control of GI hemorrhage, the site of bleeding must be accurately localized to either the upper or lower GI tract. This can be accomplished by a directed history of the bleeding, use of a nasogastric aspirate, and a rectal exam. An attempt should also be made to ascertain the volume of blood loss which has occurred.

1. History.

a. Emesis of red blood or coffee-ground material indicates that the bleeding site is within reach of the gastroscope.

b. Melena, black tarry-looking stool, usually results from a bleeding site above the ligament of Treitz. However, it may also occur from a bleeding source within the small intestine or the ascending colon.

    c. Bright red blood from the rectum may result from either an upper or lower tract source of bleeding.

        i. Rectal bleeding that results from a site within the upper GI tract represents a major hemorrhage and is usually accompanied by evidence of hemodynamic instability.

        ii. When red blood streaks the tissue paper, coats the surface of stool, or is found dripping into the toilet, the cause is either a rectal or perianal disease (e.g., hemorrhoids, rectal fissure, etc.).

        iii. Bloody stool (hematochezia) is never the result of local anorectal pathology.

2. Nasogastric Aspiration.

    a. Nasogastric (NG) aspiration should be performed whenever an upper GI tract source of bleeding is suspected, or the site of bleeding cannot be identified. However, bleeding within the proximal duodenum may be associated with a nondiagnostic NG aspirate in 15% of cases. The presence of bile-stained gastric aspirate helps to further exclude a source of bleeding within the proximal GI tract.

    b. Gastric lavage using saline or water should be performed whenever blood is discovered in the stomach, and the quantity of fluid required to clear the stomach of fresh blood should be estimated. Controversy exists as to whether the solution used for lavage should be cold (4°C) or room temperature (25°C), since cold liquids may interfere with proper coagulation. The addition of hemostatic agents to the lavage solution, such as epinephrine, norepinephrine, or thrombin, has no beneficial therapeutic effect in the control of hemorrhage.

    c. In most cases, the NG tube should be removed after completion of lavage. However, the tube should be secured in place when there is evidence of active, ongoing blood loss. This provides a means of monitoring the patient for further bleeding and can also be used to clear the stomach of blood before upper endoscopy.

3. Rectal Examination. When blood is mixed with stool, the color is dependent upon (*a*) the site of bleeding; (*b*) the volume of blood loss; and (*c*) the intestinal transit time. Black stool usually indicates bleeding from the proximal GI tract,

maroon blood/stool indicates a bleeding site within the small bowel or proximal colon, and red blood is usually the consequence of bleeding in the distal half of the large bowel.

B. Upper GI Bleeding (Fig. 3.2)
   1. Upper Endoscopy.
      a. Endoscopic examination of the upper GI tract should generally be performed in all patients with acute upper GI bleeding. The goals of upper endoscopy include:
         i. Establishing the cause of bleeding.
         ii. Identifying the actual site of blood loss when several potential lesions are present.
         iii. Making an assessment of the rate of bleeding.

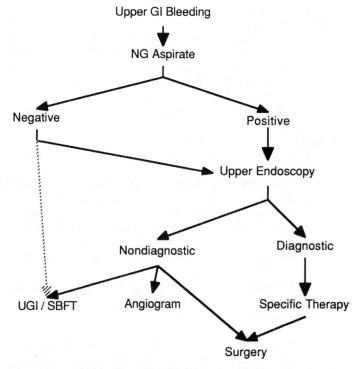

Figure 3.2.   Upper GI bleeding. Solid line, *active bleeding;* broken line, *cessation of bleeding.* SBFT, *small bowel follow through.*

        iv. Recognizing the stigmata that are associated with an increased likelihood of recurrent hemorrhage.

        v. The use of therapeutic techniques for control of bleeding.

    b. The patient should be hemodynamically stable before upper endoscopy is performed. An exception to this is the patient with life-threatening hemorrhage who may require emergency endoscopy just prior to surgery.

    c. The indications for emergency gastroscopy are:

        i. Active, uncontrolled upper GI hemorrhage.

        ii. Suspicion of bleeding esophagogastric varices.

        iii. Suspicion of aortoenteric fistula.

        iv. Application of therapeutic endoscopy for control of bleeding.

2. Upper Gastrointestinal (UGI) Series. There is little role for contrast radiography in patients with acute GI bleeding. However, the UGI series is often helpful in patients with coffee-ground emesis or melena who do not have evidence of active bleeding. The advantages of this procedure include (a) an ability to visualize the entire small intestine; (b) the assessment of extramucosal disease of the GI tract; and (c) greater safety.

3. Angiography is indicated:

    a. For the evaluation of active GI hemorrhage with a normal upper endoscopy.

    b. When there is a suspicion of an aortoenteric fistula.

    c. As an alternative to surgery, for therapeutic control of continued GI hemorrhage in high-risk patients who are bleeding from an ulcer, gastritis, or a Mallory-Weiss tear.

4. Surgery should be considered:

    a. When blood loss exceeds 4 units in a single 24-hour period.

    b. When there is significant rebleeding after an initial period of stabilization.

C. Lower GI Bleeding (Fig. 3.3)

1. Sigmoidoscopy.

    a. Sigmoidoscopy should be part of the initial evaluation in all patients with suspected lower GI bleeding. While either the rigid or the flexible sigmoidoscope can be used to examine patients with rectal bleeding, the rigid proctoscope has a larger working channel, which permits better visualization.

   b. The purpose of this examination is to distinguish perirectal bleeding (i.e., hemorrhoids, colitis, rectal neoplasm) from a more proximal site of blood loss.

2. Bleeding Scan.

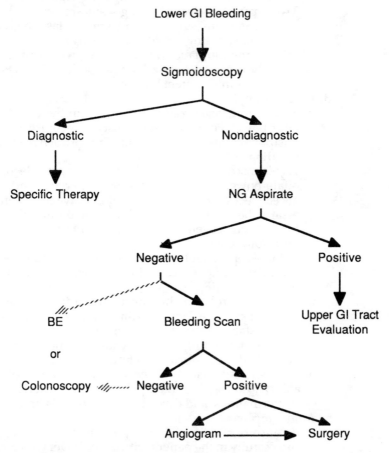

Figure 3.3.   Lower GI bleeding. Solid line, *active bleeding;* broken line, *cessation of bleeding.*

    a. The nuclear bleeding scan is a sensitive indicator of lower GI bleeding, and is capable of detecting blood loss at a rate of 0.1–0.5 ml/minute or greater.

    b. The bleeding scan can be used to:

        i. Demonstrate the presence of active or episodic bleeding.

        ii. Localize the site of bleeding to the right or left colon.

    c. Two types of nuclear bleeding scans are available:

        i. Technetium sulfur-colloid scan, a fast method of demonstrating the site of bleeding.

        ii. Technetium-labeled red cell scan, which can be serially repeated over a 24-hour period. This test can detect intermittent bleeding.

3. Colonoscopy.

    a. Endoscopic visualization is difficult in the blood-filled large bowel. For this reason, most endoscopists prefer to postpone colonoscopy in the patient with active lower GI bleeding.

    b. If colonoscopy is attempted during an acute bleed, adequate bowel preparation can be achieved using a balanced electrolyte solution for colonic lavage. When necessary, the solution can be administered through an NG tube. Within several hours, the patient can be prepared for colonoscopy.

    c. Colonoscopy should be accomplished within the first several days after the cessation of a lower GI hemorrhage.

4. Barium Enema (BE).

    a. There is no role for this procedure in the patient with active bleeding. When bleeding has ceased and the patient is stable, either BE or colonoscopy should be performed, depending on the availability of experienced individuals to perform each test.

    b. A BE will successfully detect most colon cancers, but its ability to recognize small polyps, colitis, arteriovenous malformations, and diverticular bleeding is limited.

5. Angiography.

    a. Because of the limited ability to perform colonoscopy successfully in the patient with active lower GI bleeding, angiographic localization of lower intestinal bleeding has greater importance.

    b. The rate of bleeding must be at least 1–2 ml/minute in order for the angiogram to demonstrate the site of bleeding. It is often helpful to perform a nuclear bleeding scan prior to angiography. If the scan is normal, angiography will most likely not be of value.

    c. Angiography is an important diagnostic tool when surgery is contemplated. Localization of the bleeding site to the right or left colon will direct the surgeon's attention to the proper part of the bowel.

    d. Therapeutic angiography, using either selective intraarterial vasopressin, or selective embolism, is an important modality for the control of lower GI hemorrhage.

  6. Surgery should be considered only in cases of life-threatening hemorrhage. Whenever possible, the site of bleeding should be localized to the right or left side of the colon.

UPPER GASTROINTESTINAL TRACT BLEEDING (Table 3.1)

I. Definition

  A. Bleeding Proximal to the Ligament of Treitz

  B. Two Degrees of Bleeding

    1. Massive Bleeding. Requires 4 or more units of blood within 12 hours.

      a. Presents as hematochezia as well as hematemesis. If present together, the mortality approaches 30%.

      b. Hemodynamic instability with orthostatic hypotension or shock.

      c. Differential diagnosis includes esophageal varices, peptic ulcer disease, gastritis, Mallory-Weiss tear, and aorto-enteric fistula.

    2. Low-Grade Bleeding.

      a. May present acutely with hematemesis, emesis of coffee-ground material, melena, occult bleeding, or symptoms of anemia.

      b. No signs of hemodynamic instability.

      c. Differential diagnosis includes esophagitis, gastritis, peptic ulcer disease, gastric vascular telangiectasias, or GI neoplasms.

Table 3.1.
Causes of Upper GI Bleeding

Esophagitis
Mallory-Weiss tear
Esophageal varices
Gastritis
Gastric ulcer
Arteriovenous malformation
Duodenitis
Duodenal ulcer
Aortoduodenal fistula
Marginal ulcer
Ménétrier's disease
Tumors
  Leiomyoma
  Leiomyosarcoma
  Adenocarcinoma
  Squamous carcinoma
  Lymphoma

II. Esophageal Varices

A. Pathogenesis
1. Dilated submucosal veins in the esophagus resulting from obstruction of the portal vein and back pressure on the gastric veins.
2. Portal hypertension is usually secondary to intrahepatic disease (e.g., cirrhosis) but may also result from extrahepatic disorders (portal vein thrombosis, Budd-Chiari syndrome).
3. Portal hypertension is defined as pressures in excess of 30 cm of saline. Normal pressure is 10–15 cm of saline.
4. In the United States, varices are most commonly a result of alcoholic liver disease.
B. Clinical Characteristics
1. Painless, massive hemorrhage in a patient with known liver disease.
2. Physical examination may reveal stigmata of chronic liver disease (see above).
3. Patients with liver disease may have an associated coagulopathy and/or thrombocytopenia.

4. The risk of variceal bleeding is most directly related to the size of the varix.
5. Overall prognosis is poor:
   a. One-third die during initial hospitalization.
   b. One-third die within the first 6 weeks after hemorrhage.
   c. One-third die during the 1st year after bleeding.
C. Diagnosis
   1. Upper endoscopy is the most important diagnostic modality in the assessment of a bleeding patient in whom there is either a history of alcohol abuse or evidence of chronic liver disease.
      a. The endoscopic diagnosis of bleeding esophageal varices is made either when active bleeding from a varix is seen, or when varices are found and no other potential source of hemorrhage is present.
      b. Endoscopically, a large distended varix with an area of reddened mucosa, the "red wale" sign, indicates a high risk of variceal hemorrhage.
   2. Varices can be demonstrated radiographically by barium swallow, using thick barium paste.
   3. Portal venous collaterals may be incidentally found on abdominal ultrasound.
D. Management (Fig. 3.4 and Table 3.2)
   1. General Measures.
      a. Limit intravenous fluids except blood products to prevent the accumulation of ascites.
      b. Fresh frozen plasma may be necessary to correct the coagulopathy.
      c. Platelet transfusion is rarely required, although these patients are moderately thrombocytopenic.
   2. Vasopressin. Acts to vasoconstrict the mesenteric arteries, leading to the lowering of portal pressures.
      a. Controlled trials have failed to demonstrate efficacy in management of variceal hemorrhage.
      b. When necessary, should be given intravenously.
      c. Dosage.
         i. Bolus of 20 units administered over 20 minutes.
         ii. Continuous intravenous infusion at a rate of 0.2–0.6 units/minute.
      c. Administration.

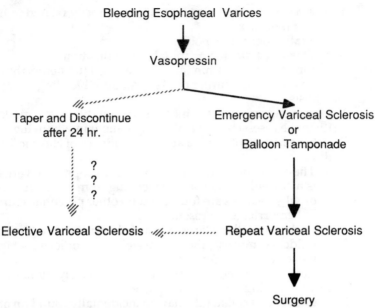

Figure 3.4. Bleeding esophageal varices. Solid line, *active bleeding;* broken line, *cessation of bleeding.*

      i. Prepare by adding 250 units of vasopressin to 250 ml of 5% dextrose in water (1 unit/ml) and administer via an infusion pump.

     ii. Should be used in the intensive care unit with the patient on cardiac monitor.

   iii. When bleeding has ceased, vasopressin should be tapered and discontinued over 12–24 hours.

  d. Complications.

      i. Cardiotoxicity: Arrhythmias, coronary artery vasoconstriction, myocardial infarction, congestive heart failure.

     ii. Peripheral vasoconstriction with gangrene of digits.

3. Somatostatin. May be used to lower portal pressure. Controlled trials using this agent are now in progress.

Table 3.2.
GI Hemorrhage—Pharmacologic Agents

Antacids		
	Acid-Neutralizing Capacity (mEq/5 ml)	Dosage
Amphojel	7	For most antacid for-
Maalox TC	21	mulas, dosage is
Mylanta II	18	15–30 ml every hr;
Riopan	9	gastric pH should be
		more than 3.5

Histamine-2 Receptor Antagonists		
	Dosage	Adverse Effects
Cimetidine	300 mg i.v. intermittent infusion every 6–8 hr or 900–1200 mg/24 hr by constant infusion	Confusion, lethargy Bradycardia Elevation of creatinine, and liver chemistries Impaired hepatic metabolism of other drugs

"Cytoprotective" Agent		
Sucralfate	1 gram p.o. every 6 hr	Constipation May interfere with absorption of other drugs

Vasoconstrictor Agent		
Vasopressin	Intravenous: 20 units (U) loading dose over 20–30 min, then 0.2–0.6 U/min by constant infusion Intraarterial: 0.1 U/m, maximum of 0.4 U/min for 12–24 hr, then taper and discontinue over next 12 hr	Myocardial ischemia, arrhythmias, hypertension Oliguria Hyponatremia Peripheral vasoconstriction Intestinal infarction

4. Balloon Tamponade (Sengstaken-Blakemore Tube).
   a. A triple-lumen tube that can produce direct compression of varices using inflatable balloons.
   b. Two balloons:
      i. Gastric balloon. Filled with 300 ml of air. The tube should be positioned properly within the stomach and its position checked radiographically before it is inflated. The tube is positioned at the esophago-gastric junction compressing the coronary veins.
      ii. Esophageal balloon. Inflated with air to 15–30 mm Hg using a pressure gauge. The esphageal balloon should always be inflated after the gastric balloon is filled. The esophageal balloon should be deflated for 30 minutes every 12 hours. Prolonged inflation for more than 24 hours increases the risk of esophageal ischemia and perforation.
   c. As the tube exits the nose, it is held taut by tying it at any one of several locations: a sponge held at the nares, football helmet worn by the patient, or a 2-pound weight suspended over the top of an orthopedic bed.
   d. An NG tube should be inserted to remove secretions that pool above the esophageal balloon.
   e. Usually advisable to intubate patient prior to use of balloon tamponade to protect the airway.
   f. Successfully controls hemorrhage in 85% of cases, although the rate of rebleeding following decompression of balloons is very high (65%).
5. Endoscopic Variceal Sclerotherapy (EVS).
   a. Endoscopic injection of a sclerosing agent into or around the varices to control hemorrhage.
   b. Acutely, cessation of variceal bleeding results from edema and compression of the veins.
   c. The long-term effect of sclerotherapy is scarring and fibrosis of the esophageal wall, providing greater resistance to variceal rupture.
   d. EVS will successfully control acute variceal bleeding in up to 98% of cases.
   e. Long-term results of EVS remain unproven. While several studies report improved survival of patients with

       bleeding varices treated with EVS, this has not been confirmed by others.

    f. Prophylactic EVS has not been proven to be helpful for nonbleeding varices.

    g. Complications.

       i. Early (< 1 week): fever, bacteremia, pleural effusion, pneumonia, esophageal ulceration, mediastinitis, dysphagia, rebleeding.

      ii. Late (>1 week): esophageal stricture, gastroduodenal varices.

6. Portosystemic Shunt Surgery.

    a. Emergency Surgery. Rarely indicated, since the mortality exceeds 75% in the patient with ongoing variceal bleeding.

    b. Elective Surgery.

       i. Patients who have had previous bleeding from varices.

      ii. Prevents recurrent hemorrhage, although the mortality remains the same due to death from sepsis and liver failure.

7. Propranolol. Although it reduces portal vein blood flow and portal pressures, has not been proven to be successful in the long-term prevention of recurrent variceal bleeding.

III. Esophagitis

A. Pathogenesis

   1. Peptic. Reduced lower esophageal sphincter pressure (LES), spontaneous relaxation of the LES, diminished esophageal acid clearance, delayed gastric emptying.

   2. Infection. Cytomegalovirus, *Candida albicans*, herpes simplex.

   3. Toxins. Alcohol, caustic substances, various medications including tetracycline, quinidine, potassium.

B. Clinical Characteristics

Symptoms of esophagitis include heartburn, chest pain, odynophagia, dysphagia, hoarseness of voice, pulmonary aspiration, regurgitation, and waterbrash.

C. Diagnosis

   1. Tests of the Potential for Reflux.

    a. Barium swallow, demonstrating hiatus hernia.

    b. Esophageal manometry, demonstrating diminished LES pressures and impaired esophageal peristalsis.

2. Tests Showing Evidence of Muscosal Damage.

    a. Barium swallow, showing esophagitis.

    b. Acid perfusion test (Bernstein test), reproducing the patient's symptoms.

3. Tests Demonstrating Gastroesophageal Reflux.

    a. Gastroesophageal scintigraphy.

    b. Esophageal pH monitoring.

D. Management

  1. Eliminate the offending agent, when possible.

  2. Administer histamine-2 (H-2) receptor antagonists and antacids.

  3. Acute bleeding will usually cease spontaneously without specific intervention.

  4. See Chapter 2 for therapy of esophagitis.

IV. Mallory-Weiss Tear

A. Pathogenesis

  1. Arterial bleeding due to a mucosal tear at the esophagogastric junction.

  2. Usually associated with a hiatus hernia.

B. Clinical Characteristics

  1. History of vomiting or retching found in 85% of patients with this disorder.

  2. Most cases found in patients with history of alcohol abuse.

  3. In most cases, the bleeding subsides spontaneously without significant blood loss.

C. Diagnosis

Endoscopically, a linear tear is found at the esophagogastric junction. At times, it may be difficult to visualize a break in the mucosa, but active bleeding from this site will be seen.

D. Management

  1. Most bleeding will stop spontaneously within 24–48 hours without any intervention.

  2. Profuse bleeding due to this lesion may be controlled endoscopically with injection therapy, laser, or coagulating contact probe.

    3. Intraarterial vasopressin is also effective for patients with uncontrolled hemorrhage.

    4. Surgical intervention may be required for the rare patient with exsanguinating hemorrhage due to this lesion.

V. Gastritis

A. Pathogenesis
1. Erosion of gastric mucosa by an irritant material (e.g., gastric acid, bile reflux, medications, toxins).
2. Impairment of natural defenses (cytoprotection) is as important as the presence of the irritant.

B. Clinical Characteristics
1. Usually painless bleeding.
2. Suspect in the patient with a history of ingesting aspirin or other gastric irritants, or any patient who is acutely ill.

C. Diagnosis
In the patient with acute GI bleeding, the diagnosis is best made by upper endoscopy. When the bleeding is minimal, radiographic examination of the stomach may establish the diagnosis.

D. Management
1. Prevention.
    a. In the acutely ill patient, the gastric pH should be titrated above 3.5 using antacids and/or H-2 receptor antagonists.
    b. All patients in an intensive care unit should be treated with either H-2 blockers or antacids.
2. Elimination of the contributing pathogenetic factors (medication, sepsis, diabetic ketoacidosis, etc.).
3. Antacids administered round the clock to maintain gastric pH greater than 3.5.
4. H-2 antagonists have not been proven to be of value in control of hemorrhage.
5. Selective intraarterial vasopressin is successful for control of severe hemorrhage in 85% of cases.
6. Endoscopic hemostasis usually of little value.
7. Surgery should be avoided except for exsanguinating hemorrhage. Total gastrectomy is often required.

VI. Peptic Ulcer Disease—Gastric and Duodenal Ulcer

A. Clinical Characteristics
   1. Patient may have known history of ulcer disease.
   2. Bleeding may be the presenting symptom of ulcer disease in 15% of cases.
   3. Bleeding may be accompanied by nausea, crampy abdominal pain, or diarrhea.
B. Diagnosis
   1. In the patient with active bleeding, endoscopy is the diagnostic method of choice.
      a. It is more sensitive than x-ray for diagnosis of ulcer disease.
      b. Evaluate for presence of signs that predict outcome of therapy. The presence of a sentinel clot adherent to the ulcer predicts a higher rate of early rebleeding.
      c. There is an option for therapeutic control of hemorrhage.
   2. If bleeding ceases spontaneously, an UGI series will often demonstrate the ulcer crater.
C. Management
   1. The administration of H-2 blockers will reduce the risk of rebleeding but does not help treat active bleeding.
   2. Antacids should be avoided if endoscopy is scheduled within the next several hours.
   3. Endoscopic control of hemostasis can be accomplished using a monopolar or bipolar electrode, the heater probe, or the neodymium-YAG laser.
   4. Angiography is usually not effective for control of gastroduodenal bleeding because of the profuse, dual blood supply of this region. Intraarterial vasopressin or embolization may be considered in the patient with active bleeding who is a poor risk for surgery.
   5. Surgery should be considered in the following situations:
      a. Uncontrollable hemorrhage that does not respond to vigorous fluid replacement.
      b. Continued bleeding requiring more than 5–6 units of blood over a 24-hour period.
      c. Rebleeding that requires more than 3–4 units of blood, while receiving intensive inhospital medical therapy.
      d. Rare blood type, or presence of multiple red-cell antibod-

ies, making it difficult to find compatible blood products.
  e. The elderly patient with other coexistent medical prob-
     lems.

VII. Gastric Angiodysplasia

  A. Clinical Characteristics
    1. Painless bleeding.
    2. Associated with renal disease and hereditary telangiectasia.
  B. Diagnosis and Management
    1. Diagnosis is made endoscopically.
    2. Patient may be treated endoscopically using various mo-
       dalities (e.g., heater probe, bipolar electrode, neodymium-
       YAG laser).
    3. Estrogen therapy has been used for control of recurrent
       hemorrhage from this lesion, but controlled trials are lack-
       ing.

VIII. Aortoenteric Fistula

  A. Pathogenesis
    1. Found in patients either with an abdominal aortic aneurysm
       or months to years after surgical repair of the aorta or other
       major abdominal vessels.
    2. Results from pressure and erosion at the vascular anasto-
       mosis into an adjacent segment of bowel.
    3. Most often involves the duodenum and colon, but can affect
       any intraabdominal portion of the gut.
  B. Clinical Characteristics
    1. Usually presents with massive, painless hemorrhage.
    2. Less often, bleeding may be chronic and intermittent, and
       rarely, may produce only occult blood loss.
    3. Operative mortality approximately 50%.
  C. Diagnosis and Management
    1. In the actively bleeding patient, upper endoscopy should be
       performed if the patient is hemodynamically stable. En-
       doscopy is important to document that there is no other
       cause for bleeding. It is rare for the endoscopist to visualize
       the site of an aortoenteric fistula.
    2. Angiography is the method of choice when the diagnosis is
       strongly suspected. However, a normal angiogram does not

exclude the diagnosis when no other site of bleeding has been identified.

3. Surgical exploration is required in cases of suspected aorto-enteric fistula when no other source of hemorrhage is found.

4. Treatment consists of replacing the vascular site of involvement and closing the bowel.

LOWER GASTROINTESTINAL TRACT BLEEDING (Table 3.3)

I. Upper Gastrointestinal Tract Sources

It is important to remember always that massive bleeding from the upper GI tract may manifest itself as hematochezia. Nausea, crampy abdominal pain, hyperactive bowel sounds, and hemodynamic instability are often present when such bleeding results from an upper tract source. Nasogastric aspiration should, therefore, be part of the diagnostic evaluation of any patient with red or maroon stools when sigmoidoscopy does not establish the diagno-

Table 3.3.
Causes of Lower GI Bleeding

Upper GI bleeding
Hemorrhoids
Diverticulitis
Angiodysplasia of colon
Ischemic colitis
Infectious colitis
Idiopathic inflammatory bowel disease
Aortoenteric fistula
Radiation colitis
Vasculitis
Colonic varices
Amyloidosis
Bleeding diathesis
Ulcers of colon and rectum
Tumors of large intestine
    Adenomatous polyps
    Adenocarcinoma

sis. Esophageal varices, peptic ulcer disease, gastritis, and aortoenteric fistula are the most common causes of this problem. At times, upper endoscopy may be necessary despite a clear nasogastric aspirate to exclude a bleeding site within the duodenum.

II. **Hemorrhoids**

Hemorrhoids, a submucosal plexus of veins lining the lower rectum, can be seen endoscopically in all individuals, but treatment is required only when they produce symptoms, i.e., pain or bleeding.
  A. Diagnosis
    1. External hemorrhoids are readily diagnosed by digital inspection of the perineum. They are swollen pads of tissue which may become distended due to thrombosis and produce rectal pain.
    2. Internal hemorrhoids cannot be recognized by external visual examination or by digital palpation. Their presence is best demonstrated using a beveled anoscope. The major symptom of internal hemorrhoids is rectal bleeding. The diagnosis of bleeding hemorrhoids can only be firmly established when either active bleeding from a hemorrhoid is observed, or a fresh clot is found overlying a hemorrhoid. In all other circumstances, a more thorough examination of the colon should be performed to exclude other causes of blood loss.
  B. Management
    1. The treatment of hemorrhoids (either painful or bleeding) consists of nonspecific, supportive measures: sitz baths, witch hazel compresses applied to the rectum, and either stool softeners or bulk-forming agents. In most instances, these measures are adequate to control pain or minor hemorrhage. Rectal suppositories and topical ointments have little therapeutic benefit.
    2. Although it is unusual, internal hemorrhoids occasionally result in uncontrolled bleeding. In such instances, more specific measures such as local injection of a sclerosant may be required to control blood loss.
    3. Internal hemorrhoids with recurrent bleeding can be managed by a variety of surgical techniques: injection sclero-

therapy, cryosurgery, lateral sphincterotomy, laser ablation, and hemorrhoidectomy.

III. Diverticulosis Coli

A. Pathogenesis
   1. Diverticulosis of the large bowel results from the extrusion of mucosa through the muscular layers of the intestinal wall at the site of penetrating blood vessels. This intimate relationship between mucosa and vessel accounts for one of the important complications of this disorder, intestinal bleeding.
   2. The mechanism of diverticular formation is not well understood, but it is believed to be related to segmental pressure gradients in different parts of the colon, resulting in muscular hypertrophy.
   3. Diverticula of the colon most often are found within the sigmoid but may occur in any portion of the colon. In 10% of cases, diverticulosis involves the entire colon. The bleeding most often results from diverticula within the right colon.
B. Clinical Characteristics
   1. Most individuals with diverticulosis are asymptomatic. The most common symptoms of large bowel diverticula are either abdominal pain or a change of bowel pattern.
   2. Overt GI hemorrhage occurs in about 5% of patients with diverticulosis and is usually not associated with abdominal pain. Diverticulosis rarely causes occult bleeding or iron-deficiency anemia, and an alternative explanation for these findings should be sought.
   3. Diverticular bleeding begins spontaneously. Often, the first indication of bleeding is the passage of bright red or maroon stool with clots.
   4. In most instances, the bleeding stops spontaneously. About 25% of patients will have recurrent diverticular hemorrhage, and the risk of rebleeding after the second episode is almost 50%.
C. Diagnosis
   1. The presence of diverticulosis is easily demonstrated by BE examination, but the precise site of blood loss will not be localized.

2. Endoscopically, it may be difficult to ascertain the precise site of blood loss within the colon once bleeding has ceased. The presence of either a blood clot within the lumen of a diverticulum or active bleeding from a single diverticulum is conclusive evidence of diverticular hemorrhage.

3. When patients present with massive lower GI bleeding, lower GI endoscopy may be difficult due to large amounts of blood within the colon, resulting in poor visualization. In such cases, either the nuclear bleeding scan or angiography should be performed to localize the site of bleeding more precisely.

D. Management
  1. Diverticular bleeding usually subsides spontaneously.
  2. When uncontrolled hemorrhage occurs, selective intraarterial vasopressin may effectively control bleeding. Vasopressin is administered at a rate of 0.1–0.4 units/minute for several hours and is then discontinued.
  3. Endoscopically, the heater probe, monopolar electrocautery, and laser vaporization have been used to produce hemostasis, but these techniques remain experimental for diverticular bleeding.
  4. Persistent bleeding that cannot be controlled medically requires emergency surgery. An operation should only be performed after the precise site of bleeding has been successfully demonstrated.

IV. Angiodysplasia of the Colon

A. Pathogenesis
  1. Angiodysplasia of the colon, also known as vascular ectasias or arteriovenous malformations, refers to the finding of dilated, tortuous submucosal vessels within the wall of the colon.
  2. Angiodysplasia is most often found in individuals over the age of 50 years. Although the pathogenesis of angiodysplasia is unknown, it is believed to be related to degenerative changes within the bowel that occur with aging.
  3. In about 50% of cases, angiodysplasia of the colon is associated with valvular disease of the heart, most often calcific aortic stenosis.

B. Clinical Characteristics
   1. Angiodysplasia is most often found in the cecum and ascending colon, although these lesions may be found in most parts of the GI tract.
   2. Patients with angiodysplasia do not have angiomata on the skin or within other viscera.
   3. Angiodysplasia is a major cause of lower GI bleeding in the elderly, accounting for approximately one-half of all episodes of lower intestinal hemorrhage in patients over 50 years of age.
   4. In most instances, bright red or maroon blood is seen, but about 10% of patients have only occult blood loss.
   5. Bleeding is typically of brief duration, but continued hemorrhage may occur.
C. Diagnosis
   1. Angiodysplasia of the large bowel can often be seen endoscopically. The colonoscopic appearance of vascular ectasia is a flat, spider-like cluster of tortuous submucosal vessels.
   2. In some instances, mesenteric angiography may be necessary to visualize the vascular telangiectases. The angiographic findings of angiodysplasia include (a) early venous filling of veins in the cecum and ascending colon; (b) dilated, distorted vessels within the cecum seen during the arterial phase; and (c) persistent opacification of veins in the right colon.
D. Management
   1. No treatment is required for telangiectasia of the large bowel which is incidentally discovered during routine colonoscopy.
   2. Vascular ectasias that produce bleeding can be treated endoscopically using the monopolar electrode or the heater probe, or by laser vaporization. The success rate of each of these modalities is approximately 50%.
   3. Surgery may be required when angiodysplasia results in continued hemorrhage. Colectomy should only be considered when there is persistent bleeding and the site of blood loss has been well established by angiography or technetium 99-labeled red cell scan.

V. Ischemic Colitis

A. Pathogenesis
   1. Ischemia of the large bowel occurs when there has been an interruption of blood flow to a segment of colon.
   2. Two forms of colonic ischemia exist:
      a. The *nonocclusive* form of ischemia, which occurs as a result of reduced cardiac output or interruption of the blood supply to the colon during abdominal surgery. Cardiogenic shock or cardiac arrhythmias resulting in hypotension are common settings for this form of the disease. This is the most common type of large bowel ischemia.
      b. *Occlusive* disease of the mesenteric vessels, either the arteries or veins, can also result in colonic ischemia. Thrombosis of the inferior or superior mesenteric artery, mesenteric vein thrombosis, and less commonly, emboli, can all produce ischemic colitis.

B. Clinical Characteristics
   1. Most patients with this disorder present with sudden onset of abdominal pain and bleeding. In most instances, abdominal pain precedes bleeding. Despite the intensity of this pain, the abdomen is usually soft to palpation.
   2. Two areas of the colon are particularly susceptible to ischemia, the splenic flexure and the sigmoid.
   3. Bleeding is usually self-limited and rarely requires therapeutic intervention.

C. Diagnosis
   1. The diagnosis of large bowel ischemia should be considered in any patient with hypotension, cardiac arrhythmias, recent myocardial infarction, or aortic reconstruction who presents with unexplained abdominal pain or rectal bleeding.
   2. Since ischemic colitis usually affects the left side of the colon, flexible sigmoidoscopy is often valuable in establishing the diagnosis. Extreme care should be exercised when performing endoscopy on these patients, since gangrene and perforation of the bowel are complications of this disease.
   3. Angiography should be performed in patients with sus-

pected colonic ischemia who have unremitting abdominal pain, bleeding, or signs of localized peritonitis. In nonocclusive ischemia, the angiographic demonstration of persistent vasoconstriction of the mesenteric vessels is diagnostic of this disease.

D. Management
   1. The initial treatment consists of the identification and correction of precipitating factors (i.e., low cardiac output, hypotension, volume depletion, or arrhythmias).
   2. Bowel rest and NG aspiration should be ordered. Broad-spectrum antibiotics are indicated if signs of peritonitis are present.
   3. If bleeding stops spontaneously, either BE or colonoscopy is indicated to establish the diagnosis.
   4. Uncontrolled hemorrhage requires emergency angiography both for diagnostic and therapeutic purposes.

VI. Large-Bowel Neoplasms

A. Clinical Characteristics
   1. Both benign and malignant tumors of the colon can produce blood loss. In most cases, the bleeding is minor and emergency measures are not required. Bleeding is typically episodic, usually producing red or maroon stools.
   2. Tumors less than 1 cm in diameter rarely cause detectable blood loss, and other sources of bleeding should be sought.
   3. Bleeding from large bowel neoplasms is usually painless. However, abdominal pain may result from torsion of a pedunculated polyp, producing ischemia at the head of the polyp.
B. Management
   1. Colonoscopy is the most effective method for evaluating patients with a suspected tumor of the large intestine.
   2. Colonoscopic polypectomy of sessile and pedunculated polyps is effective therapy for benign lesions. Colectomy is required for malignant tumors in which cancer cells extend into the submucosa of the bowel wall.

VII. Diseases of the Small Intestine

  A. Small Bowel Tumors
    1. Tumors of the small bowel are uncommon. The most common benign neoplasms are adenomas, leiomyomas, lipomas, and angiomas, while adenocarcinoma and lymphoma are the most frequently found malignant tumors.
    2 Most small bowel neoplasms are asymptomatic. The most common manifestation of a small bowel tumor is bleeding, either occult or overt. At times, the bleeding may be massive.
    3 The diagnosis of small bowel tumors can be a frustrating experience. Radiologic examination of the small bowel, computed tomography (CT) scan, and arteriography are all limited in their usefulness. Small bowel enteroscopy appears to be a promising diagnostic modality for discovering these lesions.
    4. Surgical resection is required for most bleeding tumors of the small intestine.
  B. Meckel's Diverticulum
    1. Results from incomplete closure of the vitelline duct, producing a blind pouch attached to the antimesenteric border of the ileum. Meckel's diverticulum usually arises within 100 cm of the ileocecal valve. It is lined by ileal mucosa in one-half of the cases, ectopic gastric mucosa in about 40%, and by duodenal, colonic, or pancreatic mucosa in the remainder.
    2. Meckel's diverticulum most often presents before the age of 2 years. it is the most common cause of lower intestinal bleeding in children, accounting for nearly one-half of all cases. Bleeding is painless, usually presenting as maroon stool.
    3. Bleeding results from peptic ulceration of ileal mucosa adjacent to functioning gastric mucosa.
    4. Barium studies of the small bowel are rarely helpful in establishing the diagnosis of Meckel's diverticulum. A scan using radiolabeled technetium, which is taken up by gastric mucosa, will detect most of the cases that have gastric mucosa.

  5. Mesenteric angiography may be helpful in patients with ongoing blood loss.
  6. Surgery is the treatment of choice for patients with bleeding from a Meckel's diverticulum.

SUGGESTED READINGS

Cello JP, Grendell JH, Crass RA, Weber TE, Trunkey DD: Endoscopic sclerotherapy versus portacaval shunt in patient with severe cirrhosis and acute variceal hemorrhage. *N Engl J Med* 316:11–15, 1987.

Eastwood GL: Endoscopic diagnosis and management of upper gastrointestinal tract bleeding. *Adv Intern Med* 30:449–470, 1984.

Kiernan PD, Pairolero PC, Hubert JP, Mucha P, Wallace RB: Aortic graft-enteric fistula. *Mayo Clin Proc* 55:731–738, 1980.

Meeroff JC: Management of massive gastrointestinal bleeding. *Hosp Pract* (Off) 21:93–98, 103–106, 1986.

Waye JD: A diagnostic approach to colon bleeding. *Mt Sinai J Med* 51:491–500, 1984.

Chapter 4

Dyspepsia and Peptic Ulcer Disease
Mark L. Chapman, M.D.

I. **Dyspepsia**

A. Definition

"Dyspepsia" is one of the most frequent problems in medical practice, and yet it has been difficult to define.

It is basically a one-word description for a complex of upper alimentary symptoms that may or may not be food-related and are generally episodic or intermittent, but which may sometimes be persistent and chronic. They include:

1. Heartburn.
2. Gastrointestinal regurgitation.
3. Dysphagia or chest pain on swallowing.
4. Anorexia, nausea, vomiting.
5. Belching, burping, flatulence, borborygmi, aerophagia.
6. Bloating.
7. Early satiety.

B. Causes

Numerous problems involving the entire gastrointestinal (GI) tract can, of course, produce "dyspepsia." Those involving the stomach and duodenum include:

1. Peptic ulcer.
   a. Chronic duodenal ulcer.
   b. Chronic gastric ulcer.
2. Gastric carcinoma.
3. Gastritis.
4. "Functional," "x-ray negative," or "nonulcer" dyspepsia:

Types of dyspepsia involving other parts of the alimentary canal include disorders of the esophagus and pancreaticobiliary tract; even 25% of patients with the irritable bowel syndrome will describe upper abdominal pain and nausea. Recent computer analysis of detailed medical histories indicate that often the cause of "dyspepsia" can be pinpointed by careful attention to specific historical information.

II. Definition and Classification of Peptic Ulcer

A. Definition
A peptic ulcer is a circumscribed discontinuity in the surface of the gastrointestinal mucosa resulting from imbalance of acid-peptic forces.
B. Classification
They can be classified by chronicity, depth, or location, i.e., gastric, duodenal, esophageal, or marginal (distal to the site of a surgically created anastomosis).

III. Epidemiology of Peptic Ulcer

Peptic ulcer has proved to be a common and costly disease, with 4 million Americans affected during any given year.
A. Frequency
The frequency of active peptic ulcer disease in the United States in 1 year (1-year-period prevalence) is 1.7%; the number of new cases per year (annual peptic ulcer incidence) is 0.29%. About 350,000 new cases of peptic ulcers occur per year in the United States.
   1. The male:female ratio for duodenal ulcer has changed from 2:1 to 1:1 over the past 20 years.
   2. Hospitalization.
      a. Hospitalization rates in the United States for peptic ulcers have been declining; they have dropped from 25.2 per 10,000 in 1965, to 16.5 per 10,000 in 1981.
      b. This reflects a decrease in hospitalization for uncomplicated cases due to increased outpatient diagnosis and treatment.
      c. There has been little or no decrease in duodenal ulcer perforations and only a slight decrease in hemorrhages.

B. Age

The incidence of duodenal ulcer rises to a plateau during middle adult life.

C. Mortality

1. The mortality rate for gastric ulcer has declined between 1962 and 1979, from 3.5 per 100,000 to 1.1 per 100,000.
2. For duodenal ulcer, the mortality rate has declined from 3.1 per 100,000 to 0.9 per 100,000.

D. Cost

The direct costs of peptic ulcers—such as hospital care, professional charges, and drugs—are $1.2 billion per year, while indirect costs for loss of work time are at least $1.5 billion per year.

E. Risk Factors

Peptic ulcer disease represents a complex interaction of multiple environmental and genetic factors which produce the disease (heterogeneity):

1. Genetic and Disease-Related Factors. Increased incidence of duodenal ulcer occurs in:
   a. First-degree relatives (parent, sibling, or child) of peptic ulcer patient, threefold increase.
   b. Identical twins of peptic ulcer patients, threefold increase; fraternal twins of peptic ulcer patient, twofold increase.
   c. Blood group O, 30% increase.
   d. Nonsecretors into saliva of ABO antigens, 50% increase.
   e. Combination of factors c and d, 150% increase.
   f. HLA-B5, -B12, and -BW35 antigens in males.
   g. α-1 antitrypsin deficiency.
   h. Type 1 multiple endocrine neoplasia (MEN) with Zollinger-Ellison (Z-E) syndrome.
   i. Systemic mastocytosis.
   j. Ulcer-tremor-nystagmus.
   k. Amyloidosis, type IV.
2. Cigarette Smoking. Cigarette smoking is associated with an increased frequency of duodenal ulcer which ranges from 33 to 110% above the rate for nonsmokers. Smoking does appear to delay healing of both duodenal and gastric ulcers.
3. Aspirin. Chronic ingestion of aspirin increases the incidence

of gastric ulcers in women, but there are no conclusive studies on duodenal ulcers.

4. Nonsteroidal Anti-Inflammatory Drugs (NSAID). Drugs such as indomethacin, ibuprofen, and others, while altering the "defensive" capability of the gastric mucosa by inhibiting prostaglandin synthesis, have not been demonstrated to produce gastric or duodenal ulcers in laboratory studies, although epidemiologic evidence associates them with increased incidence of peptic ulcers, especially in the elderly.

5. Coffee and Alcohol. Both caffeinated and decaffeinated coffees are strong stimulants of acid secretion, as are milk, beer, and soft drinks. There is considerable doubt as to an increased association of ulcer disease with either coffee or alcohol.

6. Corticosteroids. The ulcerogenic properties of corticosteroids remain generally accepted by many, although there is considerable controversy generated by conflicting studies.

7. Stress. The role of stress and personality type remains controversial, although some studies can correlate high serum pepsinogen and peptic ulcer with psychological test results that reveal intense infantile and oral dependent wishes.

IV. Pathophysiology of Peptic Ulcers

Peptic ulcers are thought to result from an imbalance between the *aggressive* forces (HCl and pepsin) that promote ulceration, and the *defensive* forces that protect the stomach (gastric mucosal barrier, gastric "mucus" barrier, HCO_3 secretion, and "cytoprotection").

A. Duodenal Ulcer
1. Hypersecretion. Fifty percent of patients with duodenal ulcer secrete excessive amounts of acid and pepsin.
   a. Duodenal ulcer (DU) stomachs have twice the number of parietal cells (2 billion) than normal, with a maximal hourly acid output of 40 mEq (twice normal).
   b. Increased parietal cell sensitivity to gastrin.
   c. Increased meal-stimulated gastrin release.
   d. Increased serum pepsinogen I concentration.
   e. Decreased acid inhibition of gastrin release.

2. Increased gastric emptying with delivery of excessive load of HCl and pepsin to duodenum.
3. Decreased duodenal defense with decreased duodenal HCO_3 secretion.

B. Gastric Ulcer
1. Decreased pyloric sphincter pressure at rest and in response to acid or fat in duodenum.
2. Increased reflux of duodenal material (bile and lysolethicin) into the stomach, which:
   a. Disrupts the gastric mucosal barrier.
   b. Leads to increased back diffusion of H^+ ions into the mucosa with subsequent histamine release, and causes mucosal damage (gastritis).
3. Chronic atrophic gastritis of antral mucosa with variable extension into acid-secreting mucosa.
4. Decreased maximal acid output in at least 50% of gastric ulcer (GU) patients, paralleling degree of involvement of acid-secreting mucosa by chronic atrophic gastritis.
5. Possible abnormalities in formation of mucous gel, which traps HCO_3 and may provide a barrier to H^+ ions through neutralization in gel layer.
6. The naturally occurring prostaglandins E_1 and E_2 in the stomach have been shown to protect the stomach from thermal and chemical damage. The mechanisms of action, i.e., increasing mucus or HCO_3 secretion, increased mucosal blood flow, or increased cell regeneration, remain unknown. The term "cyto-protection" has been used to describe the effect of these prostaglandins. Possible abnormalities in this mechanism may be present in gastric ulcer.

V. Chronic Duodenal Ulcer

A. Symptoms and History
1. Silent ulcer: Perforation and massive hemorrhage can occur from duodenal ulcers in the absence of symptoms, and endoscopic studies have revealed 15 to 44% of ulcer patients to be symptom-free.
2. About 50% of duodenal ulcer patients have a fairly characteristic "dyspeptic pattern" which consists of:

    a. Nonradiating epigastric pain described as "exaggerated hunger," "gnawing," "dull aching or burning."

    b. Pain occurs 1–3 hours after eating and is absent before breakfast.

    c. Pain frequently awakens patient at night.

    d. Pain is relieved by food, antacids, or vomiting.

    e. Clusters of daily episodes of pain occur for a few weeks, followed by longer pain-free intervals.

3. Computer analysis has shown that if the history shows the following factors, the diagnosis of chronic duodenal ulcer can approach 70%:

    a. History longer than 4 years.

    b. Pain localized to epigastrium ("pointing sign").

    c. Hypersalivation associated with pain.

    d. Family history of ulcer.

    e. Male gender.

    f. Smoking.

    g. Episodes of pain more frequent in the winter.

    h. When vomiting occurs, the patient can eat soon afterwards.

4. Reflux esophagitis is a very common disorder that can confuse. Although the heartburn in this disorder can awaken the patient at night, the symptoms usually occur immediately after meals, especially on a full stomach.

5. Other Important History.

    a. Family history: Renal stones, hyperparathyroid disease, Z-E syndrome in the MEN 1 complex.

    b. Medication history: Particularly steroids, aspirin, and NSAID.

6. Physical Examination. In uncomplicated cases, this rarely adds new information, even in the presence of epigastric tenderness.

7. Diagnostic Studies.

    a. Endoscopy. This is superior to upper GI radiology, even double-contrast studies. The recent developments of thinner (7–10 mm) endoscopes, combined with minimal sedation (intravenous Valium and Demerol) or even a topical anesthetic alone, have enhanced comfort substantially. The risk of perforation is very small, and one can identify esophagitis, gastritis, and duodenitis. Biopsies can also be obtained.

b. X-Ray. From a practical point of view, patients with symptoms referrable to the upper GI tract usually undergo radiography as the first diagnostic test, as it is cheaper and more acceptable to patients, with no risk of perforation. If the clinical response is poor, and there is a question of a correct diagnosis, endoscopy should be performed.

B. Treatment

1. Antacids.

a. Rationale. Duodenal ulcers rarely occur in the absence of acid or when the hourly maximum acid output is less than 10 mEq. Peptic activity decreases as acidity decreases; experimental ulcer formation is inhibited by antacids; and acid-reducing operations cure ulcers.

b. Pharmacology.

i. In the fasting state, antacids have only a transient intragastric buffering effect (15–20) minutes). When ingested 1 hour after a meal, they have a much more prolonged effect, about 3–4 hours; therefore, they should optimally be taken 1 and 3 hours after meals and before sleep.

ii. The buffering capacities and doses of antacids vary (Table 4.1).

iii. Diarrhea produced by magnesium-containing compounds can be lessened by alternating them with aluminum hydroxide gels.

iv. Chronic administration of calcium carbonate-containing antacids should be avoided because of hypercalcemia and Ca^{++} stimulation of acid secretion.

v. Aluminum or magnesium toxicity is unlikely in patients with normal renal function. The encephalopathy of tissue deposition of aluminum only occurs in dialysis of patients receiving $Al(OH)_3$ for control of hyperphosphatemia. Chronic use of magnesium-containing antacids is not advisable in patients with renal insufficiency.

vi. Hypophosphatemia and osteomalacia can occur in long-term use of $Al(OH)_3$, but they can also occur with short-term use in severely malnourished patients, such as alcoholics.

Table 4.1
Comparison of Antacids at at Dose of 140 mEq/Hour

Brand Name	Neutralizing Capacity (mEq H$^+$/ml antacid	Therapeutic Dose (140 mEq) (ml or # of tabs)	Composition	Na$^+$ Content (mg/day)
		Liquids (Concentrated)		
Maalox TC	4.2	33	Al(OH)$_3$ Mg(OH)$_3$	55
Titralac	4.2	33	CaCO$_3$ Glycerine	508
Delcid	4.1	34	Al(OH)$_3$ Mg(OH)$_3$	71
Mylanta II	3.6	39	AL(OH)$_3$ Mg(OH)$_3$ Simethicone	60
		Liquids (Regular)		
Camalox	3.2	44	Al(OH)$_3$ Mg(OH)$_3$ CaCO$_3$	154
Gelusil II	3.0	47	Al(OH)$_3$ Mg(OH)$_3$ Simethicone	86
Maalox Plus	2.3	61	Al(OH)$_3$ Mg(OH)$_3$ Simethicone	214
Gelusil	2.2	64	Al(OH)$_3$ Mg(OH)$_3$ Simethicone	63
Riopan Plus	1.8	78	Al(OH)$_3$ Mg(OH)$_3$ Simethicone	76
Amphojel	1.4	100	Al(OH)$_3$	980
		Tablets		
Camalox	16.7	8	Al(OH)$_3$ Mg(OH)$_3$	84
Mylanta II	11.0	13	Al(OH)$_3$ Mg(OH)$_3$ Simethicone	126

Table 4.1
Comparison of Antacids at at Dose of 140 meq/Hour*

Brand Name	Neutralizing Capacity (mEq H⁺/ml antacid)	Therapeutic Dose (140 mEq) (ml or # of tabs)	Composition	Na⁺ Content (mg/day)
		Tablets		
Tums	10.5	13	$CaCO_3$ $Al(OH)_3$ $Mg(OH)_3$	246
Riopan Plus	10.0	14	$Al(OH)_3$ $Mg(OH)_3$ Simethicone	29
Titralac	9.5	9.5	$CaCO_3$ Glycerine	32
Rolaids	6.9	6.9	$Al_2(CO_3)_3$	7420
Maalox Plus	5.7	5.7	$Al(OH)_3$ $Mg(OH)_3$ Simethicone	245
Amphojel	2.0	2.0	$Al(OH)_3$	3430

*Modified and adapted from Sleisenger MH, Fordtran JS (eds): *Gastrointestinal Disease: Pathophysiology, Diagnosis and Management.* Philadelphia, WB Saunders, 1983, p 718.

     vii. Antacids can impair absorption of tetracycline, digoxin, isoniazid (INH), iron, and cimetidine, so the dosage of antacids and those drugs should be 2 hours apart.

    viii. Low-sodium antacids obviate the problem of fluid retention in hypertension and heart disease.

2. Anticholinergics.

    a. Rationale. Anticholinergics decrease basal and stimulated gastric acid, and pepsin secretion.

    b. Pharmacology.

       i. Taken 30 minutes before food, anticholinergics inhibit meal-stimulated acid secretion by 30–50%, with a duration of 4–5 hours.

      ii. Optimal effective dose varies from patient to patient.

    iii. All have side effects to a varying degree: dry mouth, blurred vision, tachycardia, urinary retention, constipation.

iv. Should not be used in patients with urinary retention, gastric retention, or glaucoma.

v. Most useful for combination therapy in refractory duodenal ulcer disease or Z-E syndrome.

3. H-2 Receptor Antagonists.

a. Rationale. The acid-secreting parietal cell contains receptors for three naturally occurring secretory agents: acetylcholine, gastrin, and histamine. The histamine receptors are histamine-2 (H-2) receptors, as opposed to the histamine-1 (H-1) receptor sites in the bronchial tree and blood vessels. Histamine enhances the acid-secretory response at the two other receptor sites. Thus, blocking the parietal cell H-2 receptor site will decrease acid secretion in response to all stimuli. H-2 receptor antagonists (as opposed to conventional antihistamines) or H-1 receptor blockers) are proven potent inhibitors of acid secretion.

b. Pharmacology.

i. There are now four available H-2 receptor antagonists, all with slightly varying molecular configurations (Fig. 4.1).

ii. All inhibit meal-stimulated acid secretion by 80%. A nighttime dose virtually eliminates night-time acid secretion.

iii. All are primarily excreted renally. Famotidine is the slowest, with the longest duration of action.

iv. On a weight-to-weight basis, ranitidine is 5 times more potent than cimetidine, and famotidine is 3–20 times more potent than ranitidine.

v. Eighty percent of patients with duodenal ulcer will heal on one of the 4–6 week dosages shown below, as compared with about 40% of placebo-treated patients

			Total
Cimetidine	400 mg	Before lunch and at bedtime	800 mg
Rantidine	150 mg	Before lunch and at bedtime	300 mg
Famotidine	20 mg	Before lunch and at bedtime	40 mg
Nizatidine	300 mg	Before bedtime	300 mg

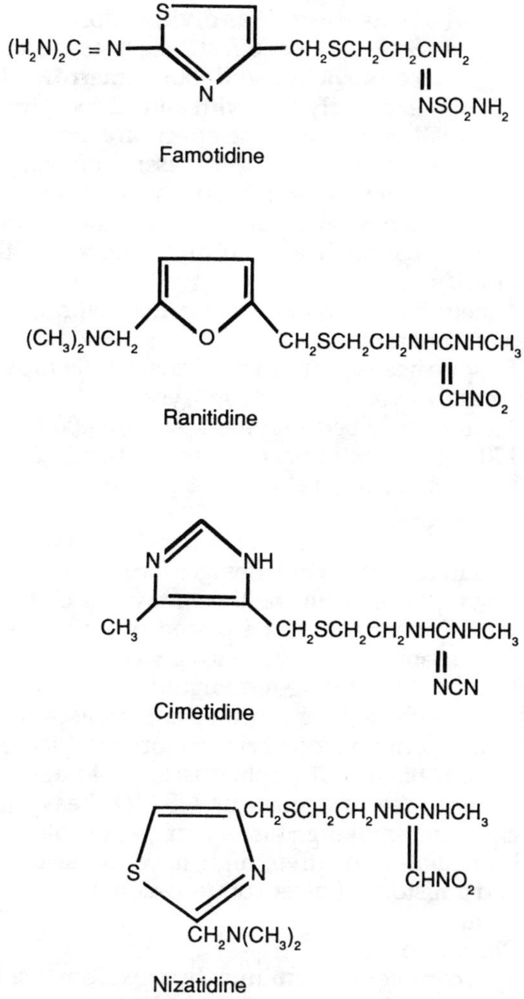

Figure 4.1. *Molecular configurations of famotidine, ranitidine, cimetidine, and nizatidine.*

Single nocturnal doses of cimetidine 800 mg, ranitidine 300 mg, and famotidine 40 mg are reported to be as effective as divided doses.

vi. Serious side effects such as nephrotoxicity, hepatotoxicity, and bone marrow depression are extremely low with all H-2 receptor antagonists.

vii. Less serious side effects are infrequently reported; they include sleepiness; confusion in the elderly; diarrhea and headache with cimetidine; muscle aches and headache with ranitidine; and constipation, headache, and dizziness with famotidine.

C. Results
1. Ninety-five percent of ulcers heal with treatment for a 3-month period.
2. Despite healing, after withdrawal of therapy, 70% of ulcers recur in 1 year, and 90% in 2 years.
3. Maintenance bedtime therapy with 400 mg of cimetidine, 150 mg of ranitidine, or 20 mg of famotidine will decrease recurrence rate to about 20% per year.

D. Recommendations
1. Treat with full-dose H-2 blockers for 6–8 weeks.
2. Continue maintenance dosages for 2 more weeks.
3. If symptoms recur, neither x-ray nor endoscopy is necessary. Patient should be placed on full-dose therapy for 6 weeks, and maintenance for 2 weeks.
4. Candidates for long-term maintenance therapy include patients with: serious concomitant diseases; four relapses per year; a combination of risk factors producing a more severe natural history of peptic disease (old age, male sex, long history, use of aspirin or NSAID, heavy alcohol intake, cigarette smoking, history of peptic ulcer disease in an immediately relative, high maximal acid output (MAO), and a history of ulcer complications).

E. Sucralfate
1. Pharmacology.
   a. A complex of aluminum hydroxide and sulfated sucrose. Because it is minimally absorbed (2–3%) from the GI tract, its activity is not due to systemic effects.
   b. Mechanism of action is precipitation in an acidic milieu forming a protective gel that binds to the material at the

base of the ulcer. Food interferes with this reaction, so sucralfate should be taken on an empty stomach.
   c. Binds to pepsin and bile salts.
   d. May stimulate release of endogenous prostaglandin E_2, enhancing "cytoprotection."
   e. May stimulate cell repair.
   f. Side effects are constipation and dry mouth.
   2. Results.
   a. One tablet taken four times daily has results comparable to appropriate antacid and H-2 receptor antagonist therapy.
   b. Maintenance therapy may be somewhat superior to H-2 receptor antagonists.
   3. Drawbacks. May interfere with absorption of orally administered digoxin, tetracycline, phenytoin, iron, and cimetidine if doses are given simultaneously.
F. Diet
   Bland diets or other controlled diets offer no advantage over regular diets in acceleration or maintenance of healing. Frequent feedings or milk ingestion can actually increase gastric acidity. Have the patient specifically avoid bothersome food.

VI. The Refractory Ulcer

The ulcer that fails to heal on a prolonged course of drug treatment, not to be confused with the ulcer that recurs after therapy is stopped. It is difficult to predict which patients will have a refractory ulcer.
A. Differential Diagnosis
   Any compliant patient who continues to have dyspeptic symptoms after 8 weeks of therapy should have gastroscopy and biopsy to exclude rare causes of ulceration in the duodenum, such as Crohn's disease, tuberculosis, lymphoma, pulmonary or secondary carcinoma, and cytomegalovirus (CMV) infection in the immunodeficient.
   1. Measure fasting plasma gastrin concentration to exclude the Zollinger-Ellison syndrome.
B. Treatment
   In the absence of clinical trials, the options are speculative:
   1. Increase dose of H-2 antagonist.
   2. Change H-2 antagonist.

3. Combination therapy with H-2 antagonist:
   a. Use of anticholinergic: Pro-Banthine (generic name: propantheline bromide) 15 mg $\frac{1}{2}$ hour before meals and at bedtime, glycopyrrolate 1–2 mg $\frac{1}{2}$ hour before meals and at bedtime, oxyphencyclimine 10 mg twice a day. There is a greater decrease in intragastric acidity with both types of drugs combined.
   b. Anticholinergic, H-2 receptor antagonist, and antacids.
   c. H-2 blockers and sucralfate: if mechanism of sucralfate is protecting the ulcer, the decreased acidity from H-2 receptor antagonist may impair binding of complex to ulcer base. If the issue is "cytoprotection," the sucralfate might be helpful.
4. Surgery.

VII. Hypergastremia

A. The Zollinger-Ellison Syndrome
   The Zollinger-Ellison (Z-E) syndrome is due to a non-β islet cell tumor of the pancreas that secretes gastrin, although extrapancreatic tumor is occasionally found in the wall of the duodenum and rarely in extra-gastrointestinal locations.
   1. Sixty percent of tumors are malignant; these produce fulminant recurrent ulcer disease, atypical ulcer location (postbulbar, jejunal) less than 25% of time time.
   2. The normal serum gastrin is 50–70 picogram per milliliter, with the upper limits of normal 150 pg/ml. Z-E patients usually have greater than 150 pg/ml and often over 1000 pg/ml. About 50% of affected patients secrete 15 mEq of hydrochloric acid per hour in the basal state, and 66% secrete 10 mEq/hr. Augmented secretory studies in Z-E usually result in a basal acid output : maximal acid output (BAO:MAO) ratio of at least 60%, as the stomach is being driven to secrete acid almost maximally in the basal state.
   3. About 70% of patients present with diarrhea.
   4. Twenty percent of patients have other endocrine adenomas, sometimes as part of the multiple endocrine neoplasia syndrome (type 1 MENS), with adenomas in the pancreas, pituitary, and adrenals.
B. Other Hypergastrinemic States

Table 4.2.
Basal Gastrin and Response to Stimulation

Disease	Basal Levels	Test Meal	Ca^{++} Infusion	Secretin Injection
Duodenal ulcer	50–70 pg/ml	Small increase in serum gastrin above normal	Small increase in serum gastrin less than 50% always	Decrease or no change in serum gastrin
Antral G-cell hyperplasia	Greater than 150 pg/ml; can be over 1000 pg/ml	Marked release of gastrin by greater than 50%	Serum gastrin may or may not increase by 50%	Serum gastrin decreases
Retained antrum	Greater than 150 mg/ml; can be over 1000 pg/ml	No change	Very small increase if at all	Serum gastrin decreases
Zollinger-Ellison syndrome	Greater than 150 pg/ml; can be over 1000 pg/ml	Little or no increase (if at all less than 50%)	Increase of serum gastrin by more than 60% or 500 pg/ml	Paradoxical increase in serum gastrin usually greater than 400 pg/ml

Other hypergastrinemic states include pernicious anemia, and less commonly, hyposecretory gastric ulcer, where the serum gastrin is not inhibited by acid entering the antrum. Additional non-Z-E states characterized by hypergastrinemia and peptic ulcer include:

1. "The retained antrum:" The antrum is inadvertently left in after subtotal gastrectomy and gastrojejunostomy and is isolated from the acid stream. Release of gastrin is no longer inhibited by low pH.
2. Hyperplasia of the gastrin cells.

C. Diagnosis
   1. Elevated serum gastrin.
   2. Secretin and less commonly Ca^{++} infusion or test meal may

aid in diagnosis of questionable cases (Table 4.2).

3. Gastric secretory studies with BAO:MAO ratios will be helpful.

D. Treatment

1. Tumor localization may be accomplished in 40% of cases with computer tomography (CT) scans, abdominal magnetic resonance imaging (MRI), angiography, and/or selective catheterization of the venous drainage of the pancreas with differential gastrin levels.

2. It is advantageous to remove an isolated malignant or potentially malignant lesion.

3. In most cases, medical therapy with large doses of H-2 receptor antagonists, as well as continuing with anticholinergics, if necessary, produces excellent control with minimal side effects.

4. Total gastrectomy is indicated if medical therapy fails. Chemotherapy can be effective in suppressing metastatic tumors.

VIII. Complications of Peptic Ulcer Disease—Bleeding

A. Hemorrhage Frequency

Bleeding is the most common complication of peptic ulcer disease, with clinically significant bleeding in 25% of cases. Occult bleeding may occur in 20–40% of cases.

1. More than 90% of all bleeding gastric and duodenal ulcerations are correctly identified by endoscopy. Endoscopy and early diagnosis have not been shown to improve patient survival or change the rate of mortality and complications. Visualization of a blood vessel at the base of an ulcer that recently bled is indicative of a higher risk (50–90%) of recurrent bleeding.

2. Despite studies to the contrary, it seems logical that when bleeding is from drug-induced gastritis, stress ulcer gastritis, Mallory-Weiss tears, esophageal or gastric varices, or rarely, ulcerating neoplasms, an accurate diagnosis can only help future management.

3. Negative nasogastric aspirates do not indicate the absence of an upper GI site for bleeding, as a tight pyloric sphincter can prevent reflux of blood into the stomach.

B. Treatment of Bleeding

1. Gastric lavage with iced saline is as likely to be detrimental as beneficial, as it may wash away clots from the bleeding site.
2. Nasogastric suction may be useful in decompressing the stomach during torrential bleeding, but its value in slow bleeding is questionable, and it can produce mucosal hemorrhage and electrolyte depletion.
3. Neither antacids nor H-2 receptor antagonists have been shown to affect the course of bleeding.
4. Vasopressin can stop bleeding from the upper GI tract, but because of side effects and lack of controlled prospective studies, its use should be restricted to desperate situations when surgical intervention is impossible.
5. Angiography with injection of autologous clot, Gel-foam, or an acrylic gel may be as useful in certain cases.
6. With the advent of endoscopic intervention, i.e., heater probe, injection therapy, bipolar coagulation, and the laser, the role of early endoscopy remains to be ascertained.

IX. Complications of Peptic Ulcer Disease—Perforation, Penetration, and Obstruction

A peptic ulcer that extends through the muscular and serosal walls of the stomach or duodenum and allows entry of luminal contents into the peritoneal cavity is said to have *perforated* (acute free perforation). If the extension is sealed by surrounding structures, i.e., lesser sac or pancreas, it is said to have *penetrated*.

A. Location
   Generally, ulcers located on the anterior wall of the duodenum, stomach, or curvatures perforate, while those located posteriorly penetrate into adjacent structures.
B. Acute Free Perforation
   1. Frequency. Five to ten percent of patients with peptic ulcer disease. Only 75% of patients have antecedent history.
   2. Symptoms. Severe epigastric pain; other symptoms include nausea, vomiting, pallor, tachycardia, diaphoresis, but rarely shock.
   3. Physical Findings. "Board-like" rigidity, rebound, tenderness, absence of both bowel sounds and liver dullness.
   4. Diagnosis. Seventy-five percent of patients will demonstrate free air in the peritoneal cavity on radiographic exam.

Extraluminal leakage may be demonstrated during ingestion of contrast material. Mild leukocytosis (10,000–15,000
cells/mm³) and normal or slightly high hematocrit may be
present. Sixteen percent of patients may have a serum amylase
exceeding 200 units, which can confuse the differential
diagnosis with pancreatitis.

5. Treatment. Most patients require surgery and closure of the
   perforation. If the patient is young and in good condition,
   without widespread peritonitis or hemorrhage, and/or has
   a strong antecedent history of ulcer problems, a definitive
   procedure can be performed. Nonoperative therapy consisting of nasogastric (NG) suction, fluid and electrolyte replacement, and broad spectrum antibiotics is rare and is
   confined to very poor surgical risks, or to prolonged presence of perforation.

6. Mortality. Ten percent of patients with acute free perforation will die.

C. Penetration

1. Location. The most frequent site of penetration from both
   duodenal and gastric ulcer is the pancreas (52.6% and 42%,
   respectively), with secondary sites being, in order of frequency, the biliary tract, the gastrohepatic omentum, and
   the liver in duodenal ulcer; and the liver in gastric ulcer.

2. Symptoms. These include referral of pain to the back, night
   distress, shift or spread of epigastric pain, distortion of the
   diurnal rhythm of distress, and refractoriness to agents
   formerly yielding relief.

3. Diagnosis. Physical exam is not helpful. A radiologic exam
   may demonstrate an accessory pocket or fistula at the site of
   an ulcer niche.

4. Treatment. Most patients with penetration or confined perforation will eventually require surgical correction even if
   they respond to modern medical programs.

D. Obstruction

1. Frequency. Obstruction occurs in slightly less than 5% of
   patients admitted to the hospital with duodenal or pyloric
   channel ulcers.

2. Etiology and Pathogenesis. Obstructing ulcers are usually
   located in the duodenum, pyloric channel, prepyloric gastric antrum, and rarely in the body of the stomach. Narrow-

ing of the lumen may result from spasm, acute inflammation and edema, muscular hypertrophy or fibrosis, and contraction of scar tissue. Most often an active peptic ulcer is present concurrently. It is unusual for scarring alone to produce obstruction. Treatment must be directed toward the active ulcer and not the obstruction alone.

3. History and Symptoms.
   a. Pyloric stenosis is the culmination of lengthy ulcer disease, and therefore occurs in older patients, most often men.
   b. Gastric stasis leads to a sensation of epigastric fullness and discomfort, increased by eating. There may be nausea and anorexia, with vigorous peristalsis causing severe pain until the stomach empties. Eventually the stomach decompensates, pain abates, and fullness becomes constant. Vomiting with relief of pain is frequent prior to decompensation and less frequent but more copious afterwards. The vomitus may contain long-retained food particles.
   c. Physical exam. In two-thirds of patients, a distinct succussion splash can be elicited. Occasionally there is visible distention. In severe cases, there is dehydration and electrolyte imbalance with neurovascular irritability.
   d. Gastric aspiration. If aspiration of the fasting stomach yields more than 100 ml of gastric contents with long-retained food, one can assume impairment of gastric emptying.
   e. Tests of gastric emptying.
      i. Saline load test: After complete emptying of the stomach, 750 ml of normal saline is rapidly infused; it is aspirated 30 minutes later. In the absence of gastric retention, less than 300 ml of fluid will be recovered.
      ii. Other tests of gastric emptying, such as the barium burger, have been supplanted by scintiscans using isotope labeling with solid food.
   f. Large overnight gastric residuals can be seen on plain abdominal films and fluoroscopy. A barium swallow can highlight modest amounts of retained materials. The greater the dilation of the stomach, the greater is the

possibility of peptic ulcer being the etiology of stenosis, due to the chronic nature of this disease. The bulk of the barium meal should be evacuated by the normal stomach in 2 hours, and none should remain after 6 hours.

g. Endoscopy may solve the differentiation between gastric outlet obstruction and gastric atony, but an obstructing lesion can be defined and biopsied even through a relatively unyielding gastric outlet.

4. Treatment.

a. Restoration of fluid and electrolyte balance, with correction of hypokalemic alkalosis with saline solution and potassium chloride.

b. Decompression of stomach: initial use of Ewald tube to remove large-caliber undigested food with gastric lavage, followed by continuous nasogastric suction. At the end of 72 hours of aspiration, a decision on further management can be made on the basis of the saline load test or measuring residual volumes. If the nighttime residual volume is greater than 200 cc 4 hours after a soft diet dinner, significant obstruction remains.

c. Intravenous cimetidine or ranitidine is given during nasogastric aspiration.

d. Peripheral or central hyperalimentation may be useful in the severely malnourished patient.

e. Surgical intervention is indicated with a long history of repeated episodes of complications and/or a failure of medical therapy.

X. Chronic Gastric Ulcer

A. Symptoms and History
The most important factors are age over 40 (higher frequency in 6th and 7th decades); female gender; frequent episodes of daily pain; pain aggravated by and not relieved by food; absence of heartburn.

B. Diagnosis.
Unlike duodenal ulcers, gastric ulcers can be malignant. Establishing a diagnosis is of marked importance.

C. Radiology
Radiologic features of benign gastric ulcers include:
1. Smooth ulcer margin.

2. The presence of Hampton's line (luminal margin of the ulcer outline by a sharply defined line representing the overhanging edge of mucosa).
3. Ulcer projects beyond gastric contour.
4. Ulcer symmetrically in inflammatory mass.
5. Obtuse angle between ulcer mound and gastric wall.

D. Endoscopy

Endoscopy should be performed on all radiographically discovered gastric ulcers considered equivocal for malignancy.
1. One out of 100 "benign" gastric ulcers is malignant.
2. During endoscopy, multiple biopsies (6–10) are obtained from the entire circumference at the edge of the ulcer. Cancer burrowing under the mucosa can be missed, as well as a small area of infiltration at the edge of the ulcer. Brush cytology may be helpful.

E. Treatment (Similar to Duodenal Ulcer)
1. Gastric ulcers heal more slowly than duodenal ulcers.
2. Forty milliequivalents of antacid, taken 1 hour and 3 hours after meals, and on retiring, is as effective as H-2 receptor antagonists.
3. When acetylsalicylic acid (ASA) drugs or NSAIDs are absolutely mandatory in a patient with a gastric ulcer, use both an antacid and H-2 blockers.
4. Gastroscopy should be repeated after 8 weeks of therapy, and repeat biopsies obtained in the absence of complete healing. In general, the ulcer should be 50% healed after 4–6 weeks of therapy, but malignant ulcers can heal incompletely.
5. If healing is not complete after 12 weeks, despite negative brushings and biopsy, surgical removal of the ulcer is recommended.
6. If a choice is made to follow a slowly healing gastric ulcer in the elderly or poor-risk patient for more than 12 weeks, frequent gastroscopy and biopsies should be performed.
7. There is no evidence to warrant a conclusion that benign gastric ulcers present a high potential origin for malignancy.

F. Recurrence

At least 50% of lesser curvature ulcers recur within 3 years and should be treated medically.

G. Complications

Complications such as bleeding and perforation are treated in the same manner as with duodenal ulcers.

XI. Acute and Chronic Gastritis

A. Erosive/Hemorrhagic Gastritis
 1. Etiology. Follows severe burns, trauma, hemorrhage, respiratory failure, sepsis.
 2. Pathology. Multiple erosions that occur primarily in the fundus of the stomach.
 3. Clinical manifestations: bleeding.
 4. Pathogenesis.
   a. H^+ ions must be present, although there is no hypersecretion.
   b. Ischemia: diminished gastric mucosal blood flow.
   c. Bile reflux.
   d. Systemic acidosis.
 5. Prevention.
   a. Correct shock from blood loss or sepsis; provide ventilatory support; correct systemic acidosis; maintain adequate nutrition.
   b. Early and aggressive neutralization of intragastric acidity. Antacid administration to keep the intragastric pH above 5.0 (at this pH, virtually all gastric acid is buffered, and the activity of the proteolytic enzyme pepsin is abolished).
   c. Use of intravenous H-2 blockers to decrease intragastric pH is probably just as effective as antacids. The choice of treatment will depend on other factors such as costs, ease of administration, renal function, presence of severe ileus, and side effects.
 6. Treatment.
   a. The same modalities as listed under "Prevention."
B. Cushing's Ulcer
 1. Etiology. Intracranial tumor, head injury, cranial surgery, intracranial infection.
 2. Pathology. Single deep ulcer may involve the esophagus, stomach, and duodenum.

3. Clinical Manifestations. Perforation as well as bleeding.
4. Pathogenesis. Marked hypersecretion of acid and pepsin due to central vagal stimulation.
5. Prevention. Aggressive neutralization of intragastric acidity.

C. Drug-Induced Gastritis
   1. Etiology. The administration of aspirin, other NSAIDs, and unrelated agents such as alcohol and bile acids. Cellular defense of "cytoprotection" may be provided by one or several of the prostaglandins (PGs) that occur naturally in the stomach (PGE$_1$ and PGE$_2$). Many agents cytotoxic to gastric mucosa inhibit endogenous formation of PG by blocking the effect of the enzyme cyclooxygenase responsible for the first step in the transformation of arachidonic acid into PG.
   2. Drug-induced ulcers are similar to stress gastritis.
   3. Clinical Presentations. Most are due to the use of aspirin or NSAID in rheumatoid arthritis or collagen vascular disease. Patients may be asymptomatic or dyspeptic, may have symptoms of chronic blood loss or, rarely, may have acute bleeding.

D. Nonerosive Nonspecific Gastritis (NNG)
   1. Definition. This is a histologic diagnosis characterized by:
      a. Involvement of the antral gland mucosa alone, fundic gland mucosa alone, or both.
      b. Disease and loss of gastric glands with intestinal metaplasia.
      c. Pseudopyloric metaplasia or replacement of fundic gland mucosa by mucus-type gland resembling the pyloric antrum.
      d. Predominantly mononuclear inflammatory infiltrate with lymphocytes and plasma cells.
   2. Clinical Manifestations. Chronic gastritis has been a synonym for NNG. Functionally, the process can vary from mild, with decreased acid secretory capacity, to severe atrophic gastritis with inability to secrete HCl and intrinsic factor. Severe NNG is often associated with antibodies to both parietal cells and intrinsic factor.

  a. Gastric ulcers are associated with antral gland gastritis and pseudopyloric metaplasia.
  b. Gastric adenocarcinoma of the body of the stomach is associated with severe extensive NNG.
  c. Pernicious anemia: Severe fundic gland atrophic gastritis is accompanied by antral gland gastritis in 20% of patients.
  d. Dyspepsia may occur in the subset of people with NNG due to mucosal inflammation.
  3. Treatment. Aside from vitamin B_{12} for pernicious anemia, no specific treatment is available.
E. Nonerosive Specific Gastritis
  These are rare and include such entities as granulomatous gastritis (Crohn's, sarcoidosis, idiopathic), Ménétrier's disease, eosinophilic gastritis, and infections such as CMV, candidiasis, and tuberculosis.
F. Helicobacter
  There are numerous reports of the organism *Campylobacter pylori* associated with gastritis; 50% of infected patients become symptomatic. It has been hypothesized that persistent gastritis and duodenal ulcers may be due to CLO infection. Healing of gastritis and ulcer with compounds (bismuth and antibiotic) bactericidal for CLO has been reported, as well as decreased incidence of ulcer relapse. The data so far appear to point to an association of CLO with some forms of gastritis and peptic ulcer, but do not strongly support the concept that this is a primary or even secondary etiologic process.

SUGGESTED READINGS

Bruckstein AH: Peptic ulcer disease: new concepts, new therapeutics. *Practical Gastroenterology* 10:74–86, 1986.

Bank S: Peptic ulcer. *Endoscopy Review* 3:74–86, 1986.

Crean GP: Symptomatic diagnosis of dyspepsia. *Practical Gastroenterology* 10:37–40, 1988.

Isenberg JI, Johannson C (eds): *Peptic Ulcer Diseases: Clinics in Gastroenterology*. Philadelphia, WB Saunders, 13(2), May, 1984.

Lam SK, Hui WM, Ng MMT: The stomach. In Gitnick G (ed): *Current Gastroenterology.* Chicago, Year Book, 1987, vol 7, pp 33–64.

Pelot D, Hollander D: Complications of peptic disease. In Bockus HL: *Gastroenterology.* Philadelphia, WB Saunders, 1985, chapter 69, pp 1155–1184.

Shuman RB, Schuster DP, Zuckerman GR: Prophylactic therapy for stress ulcer bleeding: a reappraisal. *Ann Intern Med* 106:562–581, 1987.

Weinstein WM: What is gastritis? In syllabus for AGA postgraduate course, *The Stomach and Duodenum: Consensus and Controversy,* pp 45–54, 1986.

Chapter 5

Pancreatitis
Saul G. Agus, M.D.

I. Introduction

The pancreas is a rather central organ because of its important exocrine role in the digestion and processing of food in preparation for its absorption, as well as its endocrine role, especially with respect to carbohydrate metabolism. Pancreatitis ensues when there is damage to the pancreatic acinar cell. This damage may be initiated by a variety of known and unknown causes. Following the early stages of edema, the pancreatic injury may progress to include the activation of pancreatic enzymes and thus the autodigestion that leads to pancreatic necrosis and to hemorrhage. When these factors are chronic or ongoing, the stage is set for chronic pancreatitis, which may be self-perpetuating.

II. Acute Pancreatitis

A. Pathogenesis
1. The most common cause of acute pancreatitis in this country remains alcoholism. Generally, prolonged drinking over a period of time is required, rather than binge drinking.
2. The second most common cause is biliary tract disease. This may be in the form of acute cholecystitis with or without choledocholithiasis. In addition, obstructing lesions such as tumors or strictures in the biliary tract in the region of the ampulla of Vater may cause pancreatitis.
3. In recent years, pancreatitis also has occurred commonly as a sequel to endoscopic retrograde cholangiopancreatogra-

phy (ERCP). This is especially true if there has been pancreatic acinar opacification by a pancreatic ductal injection that is excessive in pressure or volume.

4. Another known cause of pancreatitis is drug hypersensitivity. Drugs that have been implicated in the production of acute pancreatitis include: oral contraceptives, especially those with a high estrogen content; thiazide diuretics; furosemide, which is related to the thiazides; sulfonamides; tetracycline; steroids; and azathioprine. This latter drug has been used recently in the treatment of Crohn's disease as well as in the treatment of neoplasms and in transplant patients.

5. Trauma may also cause pancreatitis. This may be a direct blow to the abdomen or a consequence of an automobile accident in which the steering wheel may be pushed forcefully into the pit of the stomach.

6. Pancreatitis may result from viral infections such as mumps, infectious mononucleosis, and coxsackie virus and echovirus infections; and it may also result from infection with organisms such as *Mycoplasma pneumoniae*.

7. Pancreatitis is associated with hyperparathyroidism. In part, this may be a result of ductal calcification as well as pancreatic enzyme stimulation by hypercalcemia.

8. Pancreatitis is associated with renal insufficiency, in part because of the secondary hyperparathyroidism. There is also a high incidence of pancreatitis following renal transplantation. This may involve many factors, including renal insufficiency, antirejection drugs, vascular insufficiency, and viral infection.

9. Pancreatitis is associated with hyperlipidemia, of either the congenital or acquired type. Classically, pancreatitis has been associated with the familial hyperlipidemias of types I, IV, and V. In addition, it has been associated with the hyperlipidemia found in alcoholism.

10. Other causes include methyl alcohol poisoning, scorpion venom, and hypothermia. Several cases of pancreatitis during pregnancy have been described.

11. Even with all of these known causes, about one-third of all cases of pancreatitis are idiopathic.

B. Clinical Features
1. The dominant clinical symptom of acute pancreatitis is abdominal pain. Classically, this is constant, midepigastric pain, that radiates to the mid-back. The patient may assume a bent-forward posture in an attempt to achieve relief.
2. Nausea and vomiting are common concomitants. Intractable hiccups or retching may result. Sometimes there is actual hematemesis or melena, which can complicate the diagnostic picture.
3. Although the patient may manifest marked distress with an inability to find a comfortable position, there may be a paucity of physical findings. The most common finding is epigastric tenderness, with or without guarding.
4. Fever, tachycardia, and hypotension may be found in the acute phase. With severe hemorrhagic pancreatitis, there may be frank shock. Abdominal distention due to an associated ileus is a common finding.
5. The classic physical findings of discoloration of the periumbilical skin (Cullen's sign) or ecchymosis in the flank (Grey Turner's sign) are rare. Also unusual are peripheral signs of subcutaneous fat necrosis, although this should be looked for in all suspected cases of pancreatitis.
6. There may be pulmonary findings in up to one-third of the cases, ranging from tachypnea to focal atelectasis to unilateral or bilateral pleural effusions. An isolated left pleural effusion is highly suggestive of pancreatitis.

C. Laboratory Features
1. The hallmark of acute pancreatitis is the finding of an elevated serum amylase. In fact, it would be difficult to sustain the diagnosis in the absence of this elevation. Unfortunately, however, the elevated amylase does not have specificity with respect to the diagnosis.
2. Other conditions that may cause an elevated serum amylase are acute cholecystitis, perforated ulcer, intestinal obstruction, and intestinal ischemia. In addition, a ruptured ectopic pregnancy may be associated with an elevated amylase, presumably of tubal origin.
3. Amylase isoenzyme determination may be extremely useful in excluding nonpancreatic causes of amylase elevation. In particular, it may show parotid amylase elevation in

individuals with parotiditis or Sjögren's syndrome.

4. The amylase clearance is often increased for several days in individuals with acute pancreatitis and normal renal function. When the serum amylase is increased and the clinical picture is not suggestive of pancreatitis, calculation of the ratio of the clearance of amylase to the clearance of creatinine may be of value. In particular, this would exclude the unusual entity, macroamylasemia, as a cause of the amylase elevation. Macroamylasemia could also be excluded by checking the amylase isoenzymes.

5. The amylase:creatinine clearance ratio, which may be determined from a random urine and blood specimen, may also be elevated in other conditions, such as ketoacidosis and uremia.

6. Amylase levels greater than 1000 IU/dl usually signify gallstone pancreatitis, since alcoholic pancreatitis rarely achieves levels of this magnitude.

7. The serum lipase can be helpful when it is elevated. There are fewer false positives with the lipase than with the amylase, in that lipase is not elevated with parotiditis or macroamylasemia.

8. With acute pancreatitis, one gets elevations of the proteolytic enzymes, including trypsin, which can be measured by immunologic techniques. These tests are not readily available at the present time.

9. There are certain radiologic signs that may be very suggestive of acute pancreatitis. First of all, the chest x-ray may give some clue by demonstrating elevation of one or both diaphragms; a pleural effusion, especially left-sided; or basilar atelectasis.

10. The plain abdominal film will often given more information. Signs of a gas-filled abscess in the region of the pancreas or pancreatic calcification are usually indications of pancreatic disease. If ascites is present, one may see the "ground glass" appearance characteristic of intraabdominal fluid. In some cases, one may see an air-filled loop of bowel in the region of the pancreas, representing the so-called "sentinel loop." This probably represents localized ileus. In a similar manner, one may see the abrupt cut-off of the colon air shadow in the region of the transverse colon—

the so-called colon cut-off sign. This is nonspecific and may occur in other acute inflammatory conditions associated with ileus.

11. Ultrasound may be very helpful in demonstrating swelling and edema of the pancreas or even abscess or cyst formation. In addition, it may detect calcifications in the pancreatic ductal system. Sonography may, of course, reveal the etiology of the pancreatitis, such as gallstones. It may also reveal evidence of an aortic aneurysm or of calcifications within the aorta that may suggest an atherosclerotic etiology. Ultrasound has the advantage of being available and of being relatively inexpensive. Because it does not penetrate bowel gas, however, it may produce a technically unsatisfactory picture with acute pancreatitis. A normal ultrasound does not rule out acute pancreatitis.

12. Computed tomography (CT) scanning provides a clearer picture of the pancreas. It is generally reserved for definition of some of the complications of pancreatitis such as peudocyst formation or ductal calcification.

13. If there is ascites or a pleural effusion, aspiration of the fluid and a determination of the amylase concentration may be of diagnostic value.

D. Management

1. The clinical course of acute pancreatitis can vary from a mild, self-limited attack to a fulminant attack of hemorrhagic pancreatitis carrying a mortality greater than 50%.

2. The morbidity and mortality of acute pancreatitis is increased in older patients and in patients having their first attack of pancreatitis. A higher morbidity is associated with gallstone-related pancreatitis than with alcohol-related pancreatitis.

3. There are several factors that are considered to be of value in predicting severe pancreatitis. Severe pancreatitis has more frequent complications of abscess, necrosis, and pseudocyst, as well as a higher mortality. The indicators for severe disease, termed the *Ranson criteria*, include:
   a. Age over 55 years.
   b. Leukocytosis greater than 16,000 white blood cells/mm³.
   c. Serum glucose greater than 200 mg/dl.
   d. Lactic dehydrogenase (LDH) greater than 350 IU.

e. Aspartate aminotransferase (AST) greater than 250 IU.
f. Hematocrit drop of 10 points or greater.
g. BUN rise of 5 mg/dl or greater.
h. Arterial oxygen less than 60 mm/Hg.
i. Serum calcium less than 8.0 mg/dl.
j. Estimated retroperitoneal sequestration of fluids greater than 6 liters.

4. There is at present no specific therapy for pancreatitis. The treatment goals are to correct the fluid and electrolyte disturbances that may be present or anticipated, to treat sepsis if it is present, and to try to contain or minimize the damage caused by the release of activated pancreatic enzymes into the surrounding tissues, which causes edema and necrosis.

5. Nasogastric (NG) suction and the use of histamine-2 (H-2) inhibitors have not been shown to be of value in limiting the pancreatitis or in preventing pseudocyst formation. In the individual patient who may have gastric stasis and nausea and/or vomiting, putting the stomach "to rest" by NG suction and acid inhibition may give some symptomatic relief.

6. Prophylactic antibiotics have not been shown to be of value. Nevertheless, one should maintain a constant vigil to try to detect the complication of pancreatic abscess early and to treat it vigorously when it occurs.

7. Specific pharmacologic therapy with trypsin inhibitors has not been of value. There is interest in Europe and in the United States in the use of somatostatin and its analogues.

8. In severe cases, peritoneal lavage and even surgical exploration with the placement of multiple drains have been used with some success. This should be attempted only when the patient's course is deteriorating.

9. Theoretically, morphine should be avoided because it contributes to increasing the pressure on the sphincter of Oddi. Meperidine would therefore be a better choice.

10. A common mistake is feeding the patient who has pancreatitis too soon. The return of the serum amylase to normal does not necessarily indicate that the patient is ready to eat. Better indicators are the clinical findings of decreased pain and return of bowel function.

11. With gallstone pancreatitis, one has to make a clinical judgment. Many of these stones in the bile duct pass spontaneously. Some of these have been recovered in stool specimens. Some stones become impacted and may have to be removed by modern endoscopic techniques such as ERCP with basket retrieval.

12. Sometimes, in the course of acute pancreatitis, a pseudocyst may become evident either on the basis of physical exam or pseudocysts as detected by ultrasound or CT scans. Some of these pseudocysts resolve spontaneously. Indications for intervention include expansion of the pseudocyst, protracted pain, effect on adjacent organs, and evidence of infection. Approaches to the pseudocyst may include percutaneous drainage under CT or ultrasound guidance, or formal laparotomy with drainage and marsupialization of the cyst.

13. In the toxic-appearing or febrile patient, an abdominal CT scan should be performed to determine if an abscess has formed. Pancreatic abscess carries a high mortality and requires emergency surgical debridement. Often CT cannot differentiate abscess from phlegmon. The presence of air is indicative of abscess. If free fluid is seen on the CT, infection must be documented or ruled out by percutaneous fluid aspiration. Surgical drainage is mandatory if infection is found.

III. Chronic Pancreatitis

A. Pathogenesis

1. In the United States, alcohol is the major cause of chronic insult to the pancreas. In autopsy series on alcoholic men, the pathologic incidence of pancreatitis was as high as one in eight. The mechanism of the alcohol-induced injury is under active investigation but is not completely known at the present time.

2. Unsuspected biliary tract disease is another cause, albeit a less common one.

3. Traumatic injury to the pancreas, as in an automobile accident, is becoming a more common source of recurrent pain and inflammation.

4. There are some metabolic diseases that have been associ-

ated with chronic pancreatitis, such as hyperlipidemia and hyperparathyroidism.

5. There are several hereditary causes of chronic pancreatitis, including hereditary pancreatitis with or without aminoaciduria; cystic fibrosis; and hemochromatosis.

6. Pancreas divisum, especially if accompanied by stricture, may be a cause of recurrent attacks of pancreatitis. This is a controversial topic at the present.

B. Clinical and Laboratory Features

1. Chronic pancreatitis rarely gives overt signs of active inflammation such as an elevation of the serum amylase.

2. When there is enough parenchymal destruction, there is usually some clinical evidence of weight loss or maldigestion. The stool may be grossly steatorrheic.

3. With prolonged destruction of the pancreas, there is an eventual deterioration in the gland's endocrine function in relation to insulin production. Overt diabetes may result.

4. A secretin test may give a measure of the degree of pancreatic parenchymal destruction. The pancreatic output of bicarbonate and enzyme is reduced in response to a challenge dose of secretin. In later stages of chronic pancreatitis, the flow is diminished as well.

5. Radiologic findings might include pancreatic calcifications, widening or spiculation of the duodenal loop, and possible sonographic or CT scan evidence of pseudocyst formation.

6. ERCP may demonstrate some special features, such as pancreatic ductal calcifications and strictures, that are not generally revealed by other modalities. There may be associated bile duct pathology such as stone, stricture, or neoplasm. The overall size of the pancreas may be noted to be small.

7. Pancreatic scans have not yet been developed enough to be of clinical use.

C. Management

1. If maldigestion is present with symptoms of diarrhea, weight loss, or steatorrhea, pancreatic enzyme replacement therapy is indicated. Several commercial preparations are available. In order to minimize gastric digestion of the supplemental enzymes, these preparations are usually taken with meals and sometimes with a little bicarbonate.

2. Control of chronic pain often becomes a significant problem with chronic pancreatitis. The physician must zealously guard against the patient's becoming habituated or addicted to narcotic medications. This often involves intensive consultation with a pain clinic.

3. Antispasmodics, anticholinergics, and H-2 blockers have little to offer these chronically ill patients.

4. In some cases of extreme pain, celiac blockade by anesthesia may afford some relief. With successful blockade, there is danger of orthostatic hypotension. Relief by this method usually lasts for less than 6 months.

5. If a pseudocyst is present, surgical drainage is in order. The anatomic localization of the pseudocyst will determine where it should be drained.

6. In some intractable cases of chronic pancreatitis, especially where there is demonstrable ductal obstruction on ERCP, surgery may play a role. This operation may be either a fillet procedure of the ductal system or a partial pancreatectomy.

7. If there is narrowing or fibrosis at the entry point of the ampulla, endoscopic dilatation and/or stent placement may be in order.

SUGGESTED READING

Bank PA: Acute pancreatitis, when to be concerned. *Curr Concepts Gastroenterol* 12:3–16, 1988.

Chapter 6

Approach to the Patient with Liver Disease
Barbara Kapelman, M.D.

I. Overview

    A. Diagnostic Strategy
    Interpreting liver tests can be a diagnostic challenge requiring good detective work as well as good clinical judgment. Keep in mind:
      1. Which conditions the patient is likely to have, based on the history and physical examination.
      2. Whether the patient has cirrhosis.

II. History

    A. Basics
    Note age and sex.
    B. Sign and Symptoms
    Presence of right upper quadrant pain, nausea and vomiting, onset of jaundice, dark urine, light stool, pruritus, rash, joint pain, hematemesis, signs of encephalopathy, increasing abdominal girth, and pedal edema.
    C. Alcohol
    Note how much alcohol the patient drinks and for how long. Note the pattern (binge drinking, daily drinking, solitary drinking). Ask about prior "detox's" and withdrawal symptoms.
    D. Hepatitis Exposure
    Ask about past history of hepatitis and exposure to hepatitis,

including: male homosexuality or bisexuality, intravenous drug abuse (past or present), history of blood transfusion, tattoos, recent dental work, hair transplant, occupational exposure to blood (physician, nurse, lab technician, other hospital workers, dentist, dental hygienist). Ask about sexual contact or needle sharing with a person who has hepatitis, has a history of hepatitis, or falls into any of the above categories. Has the patient eaten raw shellfish recently?

E. Past Medical History
Ask about medications (present and past), prior surgery, gallstones, pancreatitis, other medical conditions, e.g., diabetes mellitus (DM), congestive heart failure (CHF), valvular heart disease, hypertriglyceridemia, Sjögren's syndrome.

F. Familial and Other Predisposing Factors
Is there a family history of liver disease, e.g., hemochromatosis, porphyria, α-1-antitrypsin deficiency? Does the patient belong to an ethnic group with a tendency to some hepatic dysfunction, e.g., sickle cell anemia in blacks? Does the patient come from an area of the world where liver disease is prevalent, e.g., hepatitis (Far East, Italy, sub-Saharan Africa), schistosomiasis (Puerto Rico, Egypt)?

G. Occupational Exposure
Is there occupational exposure to a hepatotoxin, e.g., PVC or CCl_4.

III. Physical Examination

A. General
Jaundice (implies bilirubin ≥ 3 mg/dl (50 µmol/L);*examine in natural light; if subtle, look under tongue); obesity; cachexia; "spiderman" appearance (emaciated arms and legs with ascites); hyperpigmentation; spider angiomata.

B. Hands
Palmar erythema; Dupuytren's contracture; clubbing; Terry's nails (white nails proximally with a band of normal pink at the distal edge); Muercke's lines (white lines parallel to the lunula separated by normal pink sections that remain stationary despite nail growth).

---

*Laboratory values will be given in conventional units as well as Système International (SI) units. For conversion factors, see "Checklist of Liver Tests."

C. Abdomen
   Size of liver by percussion, enlargement below right costal margin, smoothness versus nodularity, firmness, tenderness; size of spleen; presence of ascites; caput medusae. If ascites is present, can one ballott the liver and/or spleen?
D. Other Findings
   Peripheral edema; parotid enlargement; Kayser-Fleischer rings (best seen on slit-lamp examination); heart murmurs; gynecomastia; testicular atrophy; Cushingoid facies.

IV. Jaundice

Jaundice is one of the most dramatic physical findings in clinical medicine. Its presence is a good indication that pathology exists, and may give some indication of the severity of disease. It does not define etiology, however, and further investigation is necessary. In evaluating the jaundiced patient, note first whether only the bilirubin or most of the liver test results are normal. If only the bilirubin is elevated, a disorder of bilirubin metabolism is most likely. (See section entitled "Disorders of Bilirubin Metabolism.") If most of the test results are elevated to some degree, the differential diagnosis includes the entire spectrum of hepatobiliary disease. (See section entitled "Interpretation of Liver Tests.")

A. Disorders of Bilirubin Metabolism
   The differential diagnosis of jaundice is divided into unconjugated hyperbilirubinemia and conjugated hyperbilirubinemia depending on where in the process of bilirubin metabolism the defect occurs.
   1. Unconjugated Hyperbilirubinemia. The syndromes that follow cause an elevation in unconjugated bilirubin. However, the liver has a large reserve capacity to conjugate bilirubin. This fact, coupled with concomitant hepatic dysfunction, may cause mixed unconjugated/conjugated hyperbilirubinemias.
      a. Production of Bilirubin. Bilirubin is a degradation product of heme, the iron-containing nonprotein portion of the hemoglobin molecule. Between 250 and 350 mg (4000–6000 μmol) of bilirubin are produced each day.
         i. Eighty percent of the bilirubin derives from destruction of senescent red blood cells (RBCs) by the reticuloendothelial system, mainly in the spleen.

Disease process: Hemolysis causes increased production of bilirubin by shortening the RBC half-life, normally 120 days, e.g., sickle cell anemia, transfusion reaction.

ii. Twenty percent derives from ineffective erythropoeisis and nonerythroid components.

In ineffective erythropoeisis, heme from defective red-cell precursors is destroyed in the bone marrow before they can be released. *Disease process:* Pernicious anemia, thalassemia.

Nonerythroid components include heme-containing proteins other than hemoglobin, e.g., cytochrome P-450, cytochrome b_5, and catalase. *Disease process:* Anesthesia increases bilirubin formed from nonerythroid precursors. This may contribute to "postoperative jaundice."

b. Transport of Bilirubin. Unconjugated bilirubin is insoluble in an aqueous medium. In plasma it circulates bound to albumin. *Disease process:* Displacement from albumin carrier. Certain organic anions, e.g., salicylates and sulfonamides, may displace unconjugated bilirubin from the plasma carrier. In neonates this can contribute to kernicterus.

c. Hepatic Handling of Bilirubin: Steps 1 and 2. Bilirubin has no known function but must be converted to a soluble form to prevent intestinal reabsorption. The liver accomplishes this in a three-step process: uptake, conjugation, and excretion.

i. Step 1: Uptake. The liver is uniquely adapted for uptake because the sinusoidal membrane has pores that bring the bilirubin-albumin complex into the space of Disse. Carriers in the liver cell membrane bring bilirubin inside the cell, leaving albumin behind. This pathway is shared by other organic anions (bromosulfthalein (BSP), indocyanine green) but not by bile acids. Specialized proteins in the cytosol (ligandin and Z protein) bind the bilirubin and limit reflux back into plasma.

Disease process: Gilbert's syndrome (idiopathic unconjugated hyperbilirubinemia) had been considered the classic example of an uptake defect. It is suspected that a defect in conjugating enzyme may also be important or even predominant. Chronic hemolysis plays a role in many patients as well. The bilirubin level is usually <3 mg/dl (50 μmol/L) and is increased by fasting. The condition is inherited as an autosomal dominant with incomplete penetrance, and occurs in approximately 5% of the population. It is not associated with chronic liver disease.

ii. Step 2: Conjugation. Biblirubin is conjugated with glucuronic acid by the enzyme bilirubin uridine diphosphate glucuronyl transferase first to the monoglucuronide. The exact mechanism of diglucuronide formation is controversial. Bilirubin can also be conjugated with other sugars, including glucose.

Disease process: Physiologic jaundice of the newborn represents diminished conjugation due to lack of maturation of the enzyme system. Crigler-Najjar type I syndrome represents a complete lack of glucuronyl transferase, resulting in bilirubin levels of 25–48 mg/dl (428–769 μmol/L), kernicterus, and death, usually by 18 months. It is inherited as an autosomal recessive. Crigler-Najjar type II syndrome represents a partial defect of glucuronyl transferase, with bilirubin levels from 6 to 25 mg/dl (100–425 μmol/L). There is generally a good prognosis. Phenobarbital and other microsomal enzyme inducers can decrease bilirubin levels dramatically. Fasting increases the bilirubin level. The exact mode of inheritance is unclear, but it is probably an autosomal dominant with incomplete penetrance. Gilbert's syndrome (see above).

2. Conjugated Hyperbilirubinemia.
   a. Hepatic Handling of Bilirubin—Step 3: Excretion. The exact mechanism of excretion is unclear. *Disease process*: Dubin-Johnson syndrome is characterized by a reduced ability to transport organic anions (but not bile acids) from the liver cell into the bile. Jaundice may be chronic or intermittent and is usually mild, although bilirubin

levels may be as high as 6 mg/dl (100 μmol/L). Liver biopsy reveals a brown-black pigment in otherwise normal cells. Pregnancy and oral contraceptives may increase bilirubin levels. Probably inherited as an autosomal recessive. Rotor syndrome is characterized by bilirubin levels between 2 and 10 mg/dl (34–170 μmol/L), with normal excretion of cholecystographic contrast and absence of pigment on liver biopsy. There appear to be defects in hepatic uptake and storage of bilirubin as well as a putative excretory defect. Inheritance is as an autosomal recessive.

b. The Enterohepatic Circulation. Bile flows through progressively larger ducts until it reaches the common bile duct, may be stored in the gallbladder, and finally reaches the intestine. In the colon, bacteria metabolize bilirubin to a series of colorless substances collectively known as urobilinogen. These are then oxidized to brown pigments (urobilin and stercobilin). A small percentage of urobilinogen is reabsorbed and returns to the liver via the portal vein. Most of this pigment is reexcreted into bile without reconjugation.

c. Renal Handling of Bile Pigments.

i. Bilirubin. Urine does not usually contain significant amounts of bilirubin. Unconjugated bilirubin cannot be filtered because it is bound to albumin. Conjugated bilirubin can be excreted, but it is normally present in very small amounts in serum, if at all. Only in hepatobiliary disease is the serum conjugated bilirubin level elevated sufficiently to cause significant bilirubinuria. If the serum level is rising, bilirubin may appear in the urine prior to clinical jaundice. In some patients recovering from hepatobiliary disease, bilirubin may be absent in the urine while the serum level remains high, presumably due to conjugated bilirubin covalently bound to albumin (see section on bilirubin below).

V. The Interpretation of Liver Tests

The phrase "liver tests" refers to a battery of laboratory tests that are felt to be related to the liver. The term "liver function tests" is a misnomer, since only a few tests actually measure liver "function."

A. Checklist of Liver Tests
  1. Tests for Hepatocellular Injury. Hepatocellular damage (not necessarily necrosis) increases release of the following enzymes into the serum:
     a. Aspartate Aminotransferase (AST) = Serum Glutamic-Oxaloacetic Transaminase (SGOT). Present in liver, heart, kidney, and skeletal muscle. Normal range (in most laboratories): 0–40 units/L (same in SI units).
     b. Alanine Aminotransferase (ALT) = Serum Glutamic-Pyruvic Transaminase (SGPT). More is found in liver than elsewhere in the body. Normal range (in most laboratories): 0–40 units/L (same in SI units). A mnemonic: SO PLEASE (So please remember this time, I've memorized this so many times before).

AST
SGOT

SGPT
ALT
E
A
S
E

     c. Lactate Dehydrogenase (LDH). Present as five isoenzymes, the fifth of which is specific for liver, skeletal muscle, and some malignant tumors. Not useful in assessing hepatic function. Normal range: LD_5 5–30 units/L (same in SI units).
  2. Tests for Cholestasis. Cholestasis, regardless of etiology, causes the active synthesis of these enzymes with release into the serum. Cholestasis is the impairment of the normal flow of bile from the hepatocyte into the bile canaliculus, down the biliary tree, and into the duodenum. This comprehensive definition includes both extrahepatic cholestasis (mechanical biliary obstruction, "surgical jaundice") and intrahepatic cholestasis. Intrahepatic cholestasis is the ina-

bility to excrete bile into the biliary tree secondary to a defect on the cellular level, e.g., an adverse reaction to chlorpromazine. Sometimes a tumor mass within the liver mechanically blocks drainage of part of the lobe. Although this process is "intrahepatic," it is not a defect on the cellular level and is different from intrahepatic cholestasis as defined above.

a. Alkaline Phosphatase (AP). Major sources are liver and bone. Minor sources are intestine and placenta. Distinguish between liver and bone by performing a confirmatory test, e.g., γ-glutamyl transpeptidase (GGT) or 5' nucleotidase. If GGT is increased, the alkaline phosphatase is hepatic. If the GGT is normal, the alkaline phosphatase comes from bone. Alkaline phosphatase can be "fractionated" by heating to determine the heat-stable (liver) and heat-labile (bone) fractions. A mnemonic: bone burns. Normal range: Several assays are in use, with various units and varying normal ranges. Check the normal range at your hospital.

b. γ-Glutamyltransferase (GGT) = γ-Glutamyl Transpeptidase (GGTP). GGT, needed for restoration of glutathione in the liver, is a very sensitive test for disorders of liver excretory function. The kidney, pancreas and intestines contribute little. The most common cause of isolated elevated activity is alcohol use, followed by drugs (e.g., acetaminophen) and nonalcoholic fatty liver. Normal range: up to 30 units/L (same in SI units).

c. 5' Nucleotidase. Another test of hepatic excretory function used to determine if an elevated alkaline phosphatase is of hepatic or bony origin. Normal range: 0.3–2.6 Bodansky units/dl.

3. Other Liver Tests.

a. Bilirubin. (Also see section entitled "Jaundice.") Bilirubin is an end product of hemoglobin breakdown. Lipid-soluble (unconjugated) bilirubin is bound to albumin in the plasma. Once conjugated to the diglucuronide in the liver, it is water-soluble (conjugated) and excreted in the bile. Another more recently recognized fraction, conjugated bilirubin covalently bound to albumin, may be important in some patients with cholestasis. Bilirubin is elevated in hepatocellular dysfunction as well as in cholestasis and many other conditions. Total bilirubin – direct bilirubin = Indirect bilirubin. Direct and indirect bilirubin are approximations of conjugated and unconjugated bilirubin. Normal range: Total, 0.1–1.0 mg/dl (SI: 2–18 µmol/L; conversion factor 17.10); direct, 0–0.2 mg/dl (SI: 0–4 µmol/L; conversion factor 17.10).

    b. Prothrombin Time (PT). A true liver *function* test (after administration of vitamin K). May indicate liver disease on several bases (or may be unrelated, e.g., disseminated intravascular coagulation (DIC)).

       i. Hepatocellular Dysfunction. The liver normally produces all coagulation factors except factor VIII.

      ii. Cholestasis. Can cause elevated PT, since hepatic bile acids are necessary for absorption of vitamin K (as well as fats and other fat-soluble vitamins A, D, and E), and coagulation factors VI, VII, IX, and X are vitamin K-dependent. Normal range: Control ± 1 sec, e.g., 11–13 sec/12 sec.

    c. Bile Acids (Bile Salts). Bile acids (more properly bile salts, at physiologic pH) are detergent molecules formed by the metabolism of cholesterol in the liver. They are a major component of bile, in which they form micelles with cholesterol and phospholipids to aid in the absorption of dietary fat. They are absorbed in the terminal ileum via the enterohepatic circulation. Serum levels are of limited usefulness, since they are abnormal in many conditions. They may be helpful in determining if liver disease is truly present and in monitoring therapy for cholestasis (e.g., cholestyramine).

4. Viral Serology.
    a. Hepatitis A (HAV).
       i. Anti-A IgM is specific for acute infection.
      ii. Anti-A IgG implies prior infection with immunity.
    b. Hepatitis B (HBV).
       i. Hepatitis B Surface Antigen (HBsAg). Historically the "Australia antigen" of Blumberg. Present in:
         a. Acute Infection. Becomes negative in 1–12

months, occasionally is already negative when testing is initiated.

   b. Chronic Carrier State with or without Chronic Hepatitis and Cirrhosis. Becomes negative at rate of 1% of patients per year. Gene may become integrated into hepatocellular DNA.

ii. Antibody to Hepatitis B Surface Antigen (Anti-HBs). Antibody becomes detectable in serum approximately 3 months after clinical hepatitis. It can remain positive lifelong or decrease after many years. It is produced by injection of hepatitis B vaccines to afford immunity. Occasionally an isolated anti-HBs is a false positive.

iii. Hepatitis B Core Antigen (HBcAg). Core antigen is found in infected liver cells on biopsy but is not present in serum except in intact viruses coated with HBsAg.

iv. Antibody to Hepatitis B Core Antigen (Anti-HBc).

   a. Anti-HBc IgM is present during the acute phase of hepatitis B. It is a sensitive and useful test.

   b. Anti-HBc IgG can remain positive lifelong. It may be the only marker of prior hepatitis B infection. An isolated anti-HBc IgG may be a false positive.

v. "e" Antigen. It is present in patients positive for surface antigen. It is related to HBcAg. It denotes the infectious state but not necessarily chronic active hepatitis.

vi. Antibody to "e" Antigen (Anti-"e"). See "e" antigen above.

vii. Viral DNA. This is the most sensitive test of viral replication and infectivity but is not commercially available at present.

viii. DNA Polymerase. Another sensitive test of viral replication not commercially available.

   c. Non-A, Non-B Hepatitis. A serologic marker may be available soon for one form of non-A, non-B hepatitis. Its presumptive designation is hepatitis C.

d. Hepatitis D (HDV)—Delta Hepatitis. Requires HBsAg and therefore is present only in patients infected with hepatitis B.
  i. Delta Antigen. Present mainly in hepatocytic nuclei and sometimes detectable in serum early in infection.
  ii. Anti-HD.
    a. IgM. The main class of anti-HD antibodies in acute infection, where it may be transient and of low titer.
    b. IgG. High titers of anti-HD (IgG) (as well as IgM) are present in chronic infection.
e. Epstein-Barr Virus (EBV).
  i. Heterophil Test. The classic blood test for infectious mononucleosis; however, it may be negative (10–15%) in the 1st week. Antibodies to EBV are more reliable and informative.
  ii. Monospot Test. Easier, quicker, sensitive, and specific, but needs confirmation.
  iii. Antibodies to EBV Antigens. Tests are available for antibodies to a variety of EBV antigens. Interpretation of these tests can be difficult. A detailed discussion is beyond the scope of this book.
f. Cytomegalovirus (CMV).
  i. Serologic Tests. IgM antibodies are present early. Look for a fourfold rise in antibodies or persistently high titers. Remember, however, that IgG antibody titers may be high for years after infection and do not necessarily represent acute disease.
  ii. Virus Isolation. Virus may be isolated via tissue culture from blood, urine, and saliva. The latter two may represent chronic as well as acute infection, however.
g. Toxoplasmosis.
  i. Isolation of *Toxoplasma gondii*. The organism may be cultured from blood and body fluids.
  ii. Serologic Tests. The Sabin-Feldman dye test is one of several serologic tests for toxoplasmosis.

       iii. Histologic Evaluation. Tachyzoites may be demonstrable in tissue and body fluids but are difficult to recognize in liver biopsy specimens.

  5. Tests for Specific Diseases.

     a. Mitochondrial Antibody (AMA). Positive in (almost) all cases of primary biliary cirrhosis (PBC), it is occasionally positive in low titer in autoimmune chronic hepatitis and Sjögren's syndrome.

     b. Smooth Muscle Antibody (SMA). This is positive in autoimmune chronic active hepatitis. It is sometimes seen in low titer in viral hepatitis, including presumed non-A, non-B hepatitis.

     c. Ceruloplasmin. Low levels are found in Wilson's disease. Normal range: 20–35 mg/dl (SI: 200–350 mg/L; conversion factor 10).

     d. α-1-Antitrypsin. A low level is seen in α-1-antitrypsin deficiency. A low α-1-globulin on serum protein electrophoresis (SPEP) may suggest the diagnosis. Heterozygotes may have an intermediate level. Protease inhibitor (Pi) phenotyping can establish homo- or heterozygosity. Normal range: 150–350 mg/dl (SI: 1.5–3.5 g/L; conversion factor 0.01).

     e. Tests for Iron Overload. An elevated serum iron with a transferrin saturation greater than 60% suggests hemochromatosis. Iron overload may be seen in alcoholic and other liver diseases aside from genetic hemochromatosis. The ferritin level is markedly elevated in hemochromatosis, but it and serum iron may be elevated in hepatocellular necrosis as an acute phase reactant distinct from iron overload conditions.

       i. Iron. Normal range: 80–180 µg/dl (SI: 14–32 µmol/L; conversion factor 0.1791).

       ii. Total Iron-Binding Capacity (TIBC). Normal range: 250–460 µg/dl (SI: 45–82 µmol/L; conversion factor 0.1791).

       iii. Transferrin Saturation. Normal range: 20–45%.

       iv. Ferritin. Normal range: 18–300 ng/ml (SI: 18–300 µg/L; conversion factor 1.0).

    f. Tests for the Porphyrias.

i. Watson-Schwartz Test: A qualitative determination of urine porphobilinogen.
ii. Urine δ-Aminolevulinic Acid (ALA). Normal range: 1–7 mg/24 hours (SI: 8–53 μmol/day; conversion factor 7.626).
iii. Urine Porphobilinogen (PBG). Normal range: 0–2 mg/24 hours (SI: 0–8.8 μmol/day; conversion factor 4.42).
iv. Fecal Coproporphyrin. Normal range: 0–5 μg/g dry weight (SI: 0–75 nmol/g dry weight).
v. Fecal Protoporphyrin. Normal range: 0–120 μg/g dry weight (SI: 0–13 μmol/g dry weight).
vi. Urine Uroporphyrin. Normal range: 0.01–0.05 mg/24 hours (SI: 12–60 nmol/day).
vii. Urine Coproporphyrin. Normal range: <200 μg/24 hours (SI: <300 nmol/day; conversion factor 1.527).
viii. Free Erythrocyte Protoporphyrin (FEP). Normal range: 16–36 μg/dl RBC (SI: 0.28–0.64 μmol/L).

g. α-Fetoprotein (αFP, or AFP). Elevated levels are seen in primary hepatocellular carcinoma. Moderate levels (maximum 200–400 ng/ml) occur during regeneration after hepatocellular injury, e.g., hepatitis. Normal range: 0–20 ng/ml (SI: 0–20 μg/L; conversion factor 1.0).

h. Carcinoembryonic Antigen (CEA). Sometimes seen in carcinoma metastatic to liver, e.g., from colon, pancreas. Normal range: 0–2 ng/ml in nonsmokers (SI: 0–2.5 μg/L). May be higher in smokers.

i. Urine Urobilinogen. This test was used in the past to indicate total biliary obstruction. Excretion of urobilinogen into urine depends on an intact enterohepatic circulation, which would be interrupted in total biliary obstruction. Normal range: 0–4 mg/24 hours (SI: 0–6.8 μmol/day; conversion factor 1.693).

6. Other Tests That May Indicate Hepatobiliary Pathology.
a. Serum Albumin. Albumin is synthesized by hepatocytes. The serum level is influenced by hepatic function, nutrition, and abnormal losses (e.g., nephrotic syndrome). A low albumin in the face of abnormal liver tests suggests chronic rather than acute disease. Falsely low val-

ues may be seen in deeply jaundiced patients because bilirubin interferes with albumin determination. Perform an electrophoresis if the patient is jaundiced. Normal range: 3.5–5.5 g/dl (SI: 35–55 g/L; conversion factor 10).

b. Amylase. In an appropriate clinical setting, an elevated amylase suggests pancreatic disease. Several disease processes can involve both the hepatobiliary tree and the pancreas, e.g., alcohol, gallstones, hypertriglyceridemia, chronic pancreatitis with stenosis of the common bile duct, pancreatic carcinoma. Normal range: 60–180 Somogyi units/dl (SI: 13–53 nmol/L).

c. Cholesterol. Serum cholesterol may be decreased in acute hepatic inflammation and elevated in prolonged cholestasis, e.g., PBC or obstruction. Normal range: <200 mg/dl (SI: <5.2 mmol/L; conversion factor 0.02586).

d. Tests for Hemolysis. Hemolysis can increase the serum bilirubin level by flooding the hepatic capacity to handle bilirubin. After an acute hemolytic reaction, e.g., a transfusion reaction, the bilirubin will be mainly indirect. The liver has a large capacity to conjugate bilirubin, so eventually conjugated bilirubin will be present as well.

   i. Coombs Test (Direct and Indirect). Normal values: negative

   ii. Serum Haptoglobin. Normal value: 50–220 mg/dl (SI: 0.50–3.30 g/L; conversion factor 0.01).

   iii. Glucose 6-Phosphate Dehydrogenase (G6PD). Normal value: 12.1 ± 2 IU/g hemoglobin (Hb).

e. Ammonia (NH_3). Blood ammonia is a poor marker of hepatic encephalopathy. The arterial ammonia level is more accurate than the venous. Several problems are encountered in using it:

   i. Ammonia is probably not the substance that actually causes encephalopathy.

   ii. In acute hepatic encephalopathy, the NH_3 concentration may not have had time to rise. By the time it does rise, the diagnosis has been made on clinical grounds.

   iii. High levels may be encountered in cirrhotics without obvious encephalopathy, especially if a portal systemic shunt is present or if diuretics have been used. In these situations, a change in NH_3 concentration may be helpful. Normal range: 5–69 µg/dl.

f. Platelets. Low platelets may be a sign of hypersplenism secondary to splenomegaly caused by portal hypertension. Platelets may also be low because of DIC complicating liver disease. Normal range: 130,000–400,000/ml.

g. Serum Protein Electrophoresis (SPEP). "β-γ bridging" may be seen in chronic liver disease.

   i. Albumin. Normal value: 3.5–5.5 g/dl (SI: 35–55 g/L); 50–60%.

   ii. α_1-Globulin. Normal value: 0.2–0.4 g/dl (SI: 2–4 g/L); 4.2–7.2%.

   iii. α_2-Globulin. Normal value: 0.5–0.9 g/dl (SI: 5–9 g/L); 6.8–12%.

   iv. β-Globulin. Normal value: 0.6–1.1 g/dl (SI: 6–11 g/L); 9.3–15%.

   v. γ-Globulin. Normal value: 0.7–1.7 g/dl (SI: 7–17 g/L); 13–23%.

h. Macrocytosis (High MCV). Liver disease is the most common cause of larger than normal red blood cells. Alcoholism in the absence of liver disease also increases MCV. Normal value: 83–103 fL.

i. Urine Bilirubin. (See section on "Renal handling of bile pigments.") The foam test: If bilirubin is present in urine, and the specimen is shaken, the resulting foam may be yellow.

B. Three Rules and a Corollary for Interpretation of Liver Tests

1. Rule 1. Determine whether the tests for *hepatocellular injury* (AST, ALT) or the tests for *cholestasis* (alkaline phosphatase, GGT) predominate. Bilirubin is not helpful at this stage, since it can be elevated with hepatocellular injury or cholestasis. (If *only* the bilirubin is elevated, see section on "Disorders of Bilirubin Metabolism.") *Often, all the test results are abnormal to some degree.* In this case, form a tentative impression by determining which test results deviate furthest from normal.

   a. The Corollary. If *cholestasis* predominates, distinguish between *intrahepatic cholestasis* and *extrahepatic biliary obstruction.* Begin radiologic imaging with a sonogram.

Review it with the radiologist. Ask specifically about common bile duct (CBD) dilatation, the area of the pancreas, the echogenicity of the liver (evidence of metastases? fatty liver? a diffuse or a heterogenous process?). A sense of false security is sometimes engendered by a report that fails to mention CBD dilatation or a pancreatic mass when actually these areas were never seen because of technical problems or bowel gas.

i. *Extrahepatic biliary obstruction* is suggested by dilatation of the CBD and possibly the intrahepatic biliary tree. Stones are often found in the gallbladder. Their presence does not diagnose mechanical obstruction. If the symptoms are episodic, however, keep the possibility of intermittent obstruction with gallstones in mind. Bile ducts are often not dilated under these circumstances.

If the CBD is dilated, it should be imaged with contrast via endoscopic retrograde cholangiopancreatography (ERCP) or percutaneous transhepatic cholangiography (PTC). The author prefers the former, but the choice depends on the expertise available at each institution. Common causes of obstruction include: stones in the common bile duct, cancer of the pancreas or papilla of Vater, postoperative stricture of the common bile duct, sclerosing cholangitis, cholangiocarcinoma, and chronic pancreatitis.

If the CBD is not dilated, extrahepatic biliary obstruction may still be present, albeit early or partial. These situations may be suggested by the presence of fever, elevation of the white blood count, and right upper quadrant pain. If the symptoms are episodic, the obstruction may be intermittent. Clinical judgment dictates whether to perform another imaging technique. An ERCP is preferable. In most institutions, a transhepatic cholangiogram is less successful than an ERCP in the absence of dilatation. Hepatobiliary scintigraphy is sometimes useful to confirm a clinical impression of acute cholecystitis. A "HIDA" scan utilizes 99m-technetium-labeled H-methyl iminodiacetic acid. The current

Table 6.1.
Highest Activities of Aminotransferases in Various Diseases

Severe (701–10,000 units/L)	Moderate to Severe (301–700 units/L)	Moderate (151–300 units/L)	Mild (Up to 150 units/L)
Viral hepatitis (acute or relapse of chronic hepatitis, with or without fulminant hepatic failure; etiology: A, B, delta, non-A, non-B; in immunosuppressed patients: herpes simplex, CMV,* varicella-zoster)	Any condition in column 1 (mild, early, or resolving)	Any condition in columns 1 and 2 (mild, early or resolving)	Any condition in in columns 1, 2 and 3 (mild, early, or resolving)
Drug reaction (acetaminophen, halothane, INH, methyldopa)	Chronic active hepatitis (viral, autoimmune)	Alcoholic hepatitus (with or without fatty liver or cirrhosis)	Alcoholic cirrhosis
Hypotension/hypoxia (secondary to MI, GI hemorrhage, sepsis, etc.)	Acute cholecystitis (with or without common bile duct stone)	Drug reaction (chlorpromazine, erythromycin estolate)	Alcoholic fatty liver
Acute or acute on chronic passive congestion		Mononucleosis	Nonalcoholic fatty liver
Wilson's disease with fulminant hepatic failure		Syphilis	Chronic persistent hepatitis (B, non-A, non-B)
			Other viruses (rubella, rubeola, mumps, varicella-zoster)
			Biliary obstruction
			Primary biliary cirrhosis
			Sclerosing cholangitis
			Drug reaction (anabolic and contraceptive steroids)
			Chronic passive congestion
			Metastatic cancer
			Hepatocellular carcinoma
			Sepsis (without hypotension)
			Hemochromatosis
			Wilson's disease
			Granulomas (TB, sarcoid, etc.)
			Leptospirosis

*Abbreviations: CMV, cytomegalovirus; INH, isoniazid; MI, myocardial infarction; TB, tuberculosis.

agent of choice is 99m-technetium-labeled di-isopropyl iminodiacetic acid ("DISIDA"). A repeat sonogram after a week or more may show dilatation of the CBD. If a pancreatic mass is seen in the absence of CBD dilatation, a computed tomography (CT) scan of the abdomen may be done prior to ER(C)P.

ii. *Intrahepatic Cholestasis.* Consider intrahepatic cholestasis if extrahepatic biliary obstruction is ruled out. Certain clinical conditions suggest intrahepatic cholestasis immediately. Even so, it is sometimes useful to perform a sonogram to confirm the absence of mechanical obstruction. Causes of intrahepatic cholestasis include:

a. *Drug Reactions.* Drugs that are noted for causing cholestasis include chlorpromazine and anabolic and contraceptive steroids.

b. *Hepatitis.* Both alcoholic and viral hepatitis occasionally have a "cholestatic phase."

c. *Primary Biliary Cirrhosis.* This condition is most often seen in a middle-aged woman with an elevated alkaline phosphatase and possibly pruritus. Check the mitochondrial antibody and IgM (which should be elevated). A liver biopsy should confirm the diagnosis.

2. Rule 2. Note the absolute height of the results of liver tests. Table 6.1 is a general guide to the aminotransferases in various diseases. For each condition, the highest value commonly seen is noted. In mild, early, or resolving disease, values may be lower. In exceptional cases, a value may be higher. The ALT is usually higher than the AST except in liver disease secondary to alcohol or poisons. Rarely, a patient may have severe liver disease, including cirrhosis or hepatocellular carcinoma, with normal test results.

3. Rule 3. Note how the levels vary over time.

a. Aminotransferase Activities Greater than 1000. A rapid drop, e.g., 30–50 per day, suggests ischemic, toxic, or hypoxic damage as opposed to viral or drug hepatitis.

b. Aminotransferase Activities Less than 700. A rapid drop suggests relief of obstruction secondary to a gallstone.

Rarely, aminotransferase activities greater than 1000 may be secondary to gallstones. On occasion, rapid obstruction by a tumor can cause elevated aminotransferase activities, which then fall rapidly. The alkaline phosphatase level lags but eventually predominates.

SUGGESTED READINGS

The SI units are here. *JAMA* 255:2329–2339, 1986. Editorial.

Schaffner F: Tests related to the liver. In Berk JE (ed): *Bockus Gastroenterology*. Philadelphia, WB Saunders, 1985, pp 410–424.

Schiff L, Schiff ER (eds): *Diseases of the Liver*. Philadelphia, JB Lippincott, 1987.

Wright R, Millward-Sadler GH, Alberti KGMM, Karran S (eds): *Liver and Biliary Disease*. London, Ballière Tindall, WB Saunders, 1985.

Chapter 7

Gallstones and Biliary Tract Disease

Peter H. Rubin, M.D.

I. Overview

A. The Biliary Tree
The biliary tree extends from the bile canaliculus in the liver to the duodenum. It includes: bile ductules, hepatic ducts, the cystic duct, the gallbladder, the common bile duct, and the ampulla of Vater-sphincter of Oddi complex.

B. The Gallbladder
The gallbladder is normally 4 cm long and not palpable to the examining hand, but its distended fundus may be felt near the tip of the ninth costal cartilage in obstruction of the cystic or common bile duct.

C. Differential Diagnosis of Biliary Tract Disease
The biliary tree is intimately related to the liver, the pancreas, and the upper gastrointestinal (GI) tract. It is contiguous to the right diaphragm and hepatic flexure of the colon. Thus, the differential diagnosis of biliary tract disease is extensive and complex. It includes:
1. Primary liver disorders.
2. Peptic ulcer disease.
3. Coronary artery disease.
4. Diverticular colonic disease.
5. Intestinal ischemia.
6. Acute pyelonephritis.

    7. Pancreatitis.
    8. Appendicitis (especially retrocecal).
    9. Gonococcal perihepatitis (Fitz-Hugh and Curtis syndrome).
  10. Irritable bowel syndrome.
  11. Radiculopathies.
D. The Major Biliary Clinical Problems
    1. Biliary colic.
    2. Acute cholecystitis.
    3. Chronic cholecystitis.
    4. Cholangitis.
    5. Biliary tumors.
    6. Postcholecystectomy syndromes.

II. Approach to the Patient

A. History
The final common pathways of malfunction within the biliary system include: pain, fever, jaundice, acholic stools, choluria, and pruritus. None of these may be present in chronic cholecystitis or incomplete obstruction of the biliary tree, or in diabetics or otherwise immunosuppressed patients.
    1. Pain.
      a. The location is classically the right upper quadrant of the abdomen or epigastrium, with radiation to the right scapular area or back. The biliary pain may be ill-defined and present in any part of the abdomen, back, or chest. The quality and duration of pain may help to differentiate between biliary colic and acute cholecystitis (described below).
    2. Fever.
      a. Significant temperature elevation is not seen in uncomplicated biliary colic.
      b. Fever is a feature in most cases of acute cholecystitis and cholangitis.
      c. Like pain, fever may be masked in patients who are diabetics, immunosuppressed, or already on antibiotics.
    3. Jaundice.
      a. Clinically evident jaundice (serum bilirubin greater than 3 mg/100 ml), when arising from the extrahepatic bil-

iary system, bespeaks obstruction of the common bile duct or ampulla of Vater rather than simply cystic duct obstruction.

b. Jaundice is unusual in biliary colic and in uncomplicated cholecystitis but is a cardinal feature of cholangitis and obstructing tumors of the common bile duct.

4. Acholic Stools, Choluria, and Pruritus.

a. These are consequences of high-grade obstruction of the common bile duct or ampulla of Vater.

b. They may precede obvious jaundice.

B. Physical Examination

Particular attention should be given to:

1. Tenderness, fullness, and mass in the right upper quadrant of the abdomen.

a. Note should be made of whether the tenderness is to direct palpation or rebound.

b. Careful palpation may differentiate between liver and biliary structures.

c. If a mass is palpable, coexistent tenderness may be of significant diagnostic importance. As delineated in *Courvoisier's law*, a palpable, nontender gallbladder (Courvoisier gallbladder) in a patient with extrahepatic obstruction occurs more frequently when the obstruction is related to a malignancy and less commonly when obstruction is due to a stone or acute inflammation.

2. In a well-lighted room, the sclera and sublingual tissue should be examined for icterus.

3. Close inspection should be made of the skin for excoriations of the trunk and extremities due to pruritus.

4. The stool color should be observed. Light tan is typically seen in acholic stools, although it may also be seen in malabsorption and diets deficient in meats and vegetables. Grey stool (the legendary "silver stool") may be seen in ampullary carcinomas, due to the combination of acholic stools and occult blood.

C. Laboratory Features

1. Leukocytosis, with a predominance of polymorphs and segmented neutrophils, is seen in acute inflammatory states of the biliary tree but is certainly nonspecific.

    2. Elevated "liver chemistries"—aspartate aminotransferase (AST) and alanine aminotransferase (ALT) alkaline phosphatase, γ-glutamyl transpeptidase, (GGT), total bilirubin—may all be elevated in the setting of biliary tract disease. Although nonspecific, these may direct one's attention to the biliary tree, especially when the alkaline phosphatase and (GGT) are elevated out of proportion to the other markers.

    3. Serum amylase may be mildly elevated (less than three times normal) in acute cholecystitis or cholangitis. Marked elevations of amylase are much more suggestive of acute pancreatitis (most often a consequence of gallstones).

D. Specialized Studies of the Biliary System

    1. Ultrasonography. This noninvasive study has become the diagnostic screening test of choice for most biliary tract diseases. It is capable of demonstrating stones larger than a few millimeters in diameter as echogenic defects with posterior acoustic shadowing. It can also document dilatation of the extrahepatic biliary tree and thickening of the gallbladder wall.

    2. Radiography.

        a. Plain X-Ray. A radiograph without contrast will demonstrate many calcium bilirubinate gallstones, but these constitute less than 15% of gallstones in the United States. Plain x-ray can also detect air in the biliary tree, which may indicate infection or previous common duct or ampullary surgery. Occasionally, plain x-ray will demonstrate diffuse gallbladder calcification ("porcelain gallbladder") believed to be associated with high risk for gallbladder carcinoma.

        b. Oral Cholecystography. Opacification of the gallbladder by ingestion of iodinated dye, which is absorbed in the small intestine, processed and secreted by the liver, and concentrated in the gallbladder. Stones (usually radiolucent on plain x-ray) may appear as filling defects in an otherwise opacified gallbladder. Opacification will not occur if the tablets of dye are not ingested at the appropriate time, if the dye is not conducted to the small intestine or is not properly absorbed, if advanced liver dysfunction is present, if the gallbladder is obstructed, if the gallbladder is incapable of sufficiently concentrating the dye for visualization on x-ray, or if there is coexisting pancreatitis.

E. Nuclear Imaging

Scintigraphy of the biliary tree after injection with radioactive technetium compounds provides objective evidence of the patency and flow of bile within the biliary tree. It is therefore particularly useful in documenting cystic duct or common bile duct obstruction.

F. Transhepatic Cholangiography

A thin "Chiba" needle can be passed transcutaneously into the upper biliary tree and radioopaque dye injected to give a cholangiogram. It is particularly useful in dilated biliary tree for demonstrating pathology of the upper tree. It also carries the potential for therapy with drainage or stent insertion (see below).

G. Endoscopic Retrograde Cholangiography (ERCP)

This technique involves direct visualization of the ampulla of Vater with a side-viewing endoscope, followed by cannulation of the papilla and injection of radioopaque dye. This is most useful for ampullary and lower bile duct lesions. It also has potential for visualizing the pancreatic ductular system, and it too can extend to such therapeutic maneuvers as endoscopic papillotomy, stone retrieval, and stent insertion.

H. Biliary Drainage Analysis

Patients who seem likely on clinical grounds to have gallstones but whose sonograms and oral cholecystograms appear normal may be diagnosed by collecting bile from the duodenum after stimulation with cholecystokinin, and studying the collected bile by polarized microscopy, looking for typical cholesterol crystals.

III. Gallstones

Most patients with gallstones are asymptomatic and remain so. Therefore, the discovery of gallstones may not necessarily be germane to a patient's clinical condition.

A. Pathogenesis

1. Calcium bilirubinate stones arise from *precipitation* of un-

conjugated bilirubin. They may arise in either the gallbladder or in bile ducts. These are the predominant stones found in Orientals and in patients with hemolysis, hemoglobinopathies, and advanced liver disease.

2. Cholesterol stones arise by *crystalization* from bile that has become supersaturated with cholesterol. Cholesterol solubility in bile is promoted by, and is therefore directly related to, the relative concentrations of phospholipids and bile salts in the bile. The precise initiator of crystalization has not been established. These are the predominant types of gallstones in the United States, particularly prominent in women, Pima Indians, and those with terminal ileal impairment. Cholesterol stones tend to arise in gallbladder; when found in the ducts they are believed to have migrated there through the cystic duct.

B. Clinical Features

1. Gallstones are usually asymptomatic when they are confined to the gallbladder (cholelithiasis), but they are likely to cause symptoms if they obstruct bile flow in the cystic duct or common bile duct (choledocholithiasis).

2. Pain, fever, and jaundice are the important clinical sequelae of impacted gallstones.

IV. **Biliary Colic**

A. Pathogenesis

1. A struggle between the "irresistible force" (flow of bile through the cystic and common bile ducts) and the "immoveable object" (usually a stone in the cystic duct) produces *colic*—acute pain.

2. The stone has arisen within the gallbladder and attained sufficient size to prohibit its passage through the cystic duct. The clinical feature of colic is acute pain, usually localized to the epigastrium or right upper quadrant of the abdomen, sometimes with radiation to the right scapula or spine via the thoracic dermatomes. The pain often seems to occur at night, perhaps within several hours of the ingestion of a heavy meal. The proteins and fats in the meals have presumably activated cholecystokinin (CCK) release from the small bowel and thereby produced contraction of the gallbladder. The stone passes toward the cystic duct

and lodges in the neck of the gallbladder, in the cystic duct, or in the common bile duct.

3. The resulting pain is severe and persists as long as several hours.
4. Nausea and vomiting may accompany the pain, presumably from associated generalized autonomic discharge.
5. In contradistinction to acute cholecystitis (see below), no fever or chills are present.
6. The attack ends when the obstructing stone either falls back into the gallbladder or successfully traverses the duct it had been obstructing.
7. Physical examination and blood studies are nonspecific, and characteristically, after the pain subsides the patient feels entirely well.
8. Patients with a history typical of colic merit an analysis of liver chemistries, serum amylase, and complete blood cell count (CBC) to differentiate colic from acute cholecystitis, cholangitis, and pancreatitis.
9. In addition, gallbladder imaging for stones should be obtained either by ultrasonography or oral cholecystography.
10. Radionuclide scan obtained during an episode of colic would be expected to demonstrate no passage of marker from gallbladder to common bile duct, but the scan would be normal after the episode subsides.

B. Differential Diagnosis
1. Peptic esophagitis, gastritis, and ulcers can simulate colic but are often relieved by food or antacids.
2. Pancreatitis can be distinguished by its persistence, by fever, and by marked elevation of serum and/or urinary amylase.
3. Other diagnostic considerations are diverticulosis, irritable bowel syndrome, myocardial ischemia, and intestinal ischemia.
4. In a few patients after cholecystectomy, biliary colic can be simulated by sphincter of Oddi dysfunction. This is a complex and incompletely defined group of disorders, including *papillary stenosis* from stone and surgery and *biliary dyskinesia*.

C. Management
1. Attacks of biliary colic can be managed medically by advis-

ing the patient to fast, and by prescribing antispasmodics and, if necessary, analgesics.

2. Subsequent attacks can sometimes be prevented by following a low-fat diet (although this has been challenged) and ingesting anticholinergics at the outset of symptoms.
3. Strong consideration should be given to "elective interval" cholecystectomy, since further attacks of colic are likely to occur.
4. Patients with radiolucent stones (cholesterol stones) who are poor operative candidates may be considered for oral dissolution therapy with chenodeoxycholic acid or ursodeoxycholic acid, although this requires long-term therapy and is effective in only a minority of patients.
5. Unremitting pain, fever, chills, dark urine, or light stool suggest more than colic.

V. Acute Cholecystitis

A. Pathogenesis
1. Cholecystitis results from cystic duct obstruction, usually from a stone, and inflammation of the gallbladder.
2. The cause of the gallbladder inflammation has not been agreed upon but seems to involve more than the obstruction per se.
3. The gallbladder bile is usually sterile when sampled.

B. Clinical and Laboratory Features
1. The patient experiences *constant* pain in the upper abdomen, often with radiation to the right scapula.
2. Unlike colic, the pain is associated with fever, localized tenderness, and guarding (Murphy's sign), and the white blood cell count (WBC) is elevated with left shift.
3. Hepatic chemistries may be elevated severalfold, but marked elevations and deepening jaundice should suggest common duct obstruction (about 10% of cases have coexistent choledocholithiasis (and/or cholangitis) (see below).
4. The serum amylase is often moderately elevated and can complicate the differential diagnosis with acute pancreatitis.
5. There may be no symptoms or physical findings in diabetic, immunosuppressed, or elderly patients.
6. The diagnosis can be established by radionuclide scan

demonstrating obstruction of the cystic duct.
C. Differential Diagnosis
1. Acute pancreatitis. The intimate relationship between the biliary tree and the pancreas makes this a difficult differential diagnosis. In classic acute pancreatitis, however, the serum amylase elevation is significantly higher than that seen in acute uncomplicated cholecystitis.
2. A penetrating peptic ulcer.
3. Right-sided diverticulitis.
4. Acute hepatitis. Here the liver chemistry pattern characteristically is predominantly "transaminitis" rather than an "obstructive" pattern with elevated alkaline phosphatase and GGT. Transaminases can go into the 1000s with transient cholangitis as a stone passes through the CBD, but the elevation does not last more than a day or two; in hepatitis, it stays up much longer.
5. Acute appendicitis. This is particularly difficult to differentiate from cholecystitis in cases of retrocecal or upwardly directed appendices.
6. Acute pelvic inflammatory disease.
7. Intestinal ischemia.
D. Management
1. Initial treatment includes NPO, systemic antibiotics, and analgesia. In about 80% of cases the process will subside on this regimen.
2. Early surgery is indicated when:
   a. There is no significant clinical response within 48 hours.
   b. A tender mass is palpable (indicating development of empyema of the gallbladder).
   c. Deepening jaundice develops (indicating choledocholithiasis and impending cholangitis).
3. If not successfully treated, the cholecystitis can progress to gangrenous gallbladder, peritonitis, and pericholecystic abscess.

VI. Chronic Cholecystitis

A. Pathogenesis
1. Again, gallstones are usually involved in this biliary disorder.
2. There have usually been recurrent attacks of acute chole-

cystitis, and the gallbladder becomes thickened, chronically inflamed, poorly distensible, and often filled with thick bile, which may have a high calcium content ("milk of calcium bile").

B. Clinical and Laboratory Features
   1. History is less dramatic than that of either colic or acute cholecystitis. Usually, it is long-standing postprandial vague discomfort, often with eructation.
   2. Physical examination and laboratory studies are unremarkable but may include modest elevations of liver chemistries.
   3. Oral cholecystography may reveal no opacification of the gallbladder due to loss of its concentrating ability. Sonography may reveal a small, shrunken gallbladder with thickened wall or may appear normal.

C. Differential Diagnosis
   1. Irritable bowel syndrome.
   2. Peptic ulcer disease.
   3. Diverticulosis.
   4. Carcinoma of the gallbladder or pancreas.
   5. Chronic pancreatitis.

D. Management
   1. Dietary therapy with low-fat diet and symptomatic management with anticholinergics and antispasmodics may be helpful.
   2. The decision to recommend cholecystectomy is a difficult one because the nonspecific symptoms are all too often not alleviated by the surgery. In fact, the further the symptomatology deviates from classic colic and acute cholecystitis, the more chance there is for disappointing results from surgery.

VII. Cholangitis

A. Pathogenesis
   1. *Acute obstructive cholangitis* (also known as ascending cholangitis) usually arises when a stone becomes impacted in the common bile duct.
   2. Cholangitis also may arise when a duct has been narrowed by tumor or by scarring from previously passed stones or surgical trauma.

3. Rarely in western countries, the obstruction is due to ingestion of the parasitic fluke *Chonorchis sinensis*.
4. *Primary sclerosing cholangitis* is a rare disorder of the biliary tree in which fibrotic narrowing occurs. This produces cholestasis and can lead to severe hepatic impairment. This condition may be associated with inflammatory bowel disease (particularly ulcerative colitis), retroperitoneal fibrosis, and chronic thyroiditis.

B. Clinical and Laboratory Features
1. The classic clinical presentation of acute cholangitis is the triad of hectic fever, pain, and obstructive jaundice.
2. On examination, the patient is jaundiced, febrile, with rigors, and acutely ill; the upper abdomen is tender.
3. Routine laboratory tests reveal elevated WBC and liver chemistries, particularly alkaline phosphatase, GTT, and bilirubin.
4. Blood cultures may grow gram-negative or anaerobic organisms, especially *Escherichia coli*.
5. Abdominal sonography or computed tomography (CT) scan will demonstrate extrahepatic biliary dilatation and perhaps the offending calculus.
6. The extrahepatic biliary tree must be visualized to establish a diagnosis of obstructive cholangitis and to distinguish it from other entities in the differential diagnosis. For this purpose, either percutaneous cholangiography or ERCP will be necessary.
7. In primary sclerosing cholangitis, the clinical picture is usually not as dramatic as in acute obstructive cholangitis, featuring, rather, malaise, pruritus, jaundice, and low-grade fever. The diagnosis can be made by ERCP, which will demonstrate alternating areas of narrowing and dilatation of the biliary tree.

C. Differential Diagnosis
1. Acute cholecystitis and its associated differential diagnoses must be ruled out.
2. These other diagnoses can be excluded by visualization of the extrahepatic biliary tree.

D. Management
1. Therapy of acute obstructive cholangitis includes intravenous antibiotics and decompression of the biliary tree.

2. Surgical biliary decompression usually requires removal of the offending obstruction or diversion of the ductal flow by reimplantation.
3. Occasionally the diagnostic modalities of transhepatic cholangiography and ERCP can also be used therapeutically to either extract the obstructing stone or place a stent around the obstruction.
4. For primary sclerosing cholangitis there is no adequate treatment. Medical or surgical management directed at the underlying inflammatory bowel disease does not appear to affect the course of the sclerotic process. Endoscopic dilatation or stenting of narrowed segments of the ducts may be somewhat beneficial by alleviating symptoms of cholestasis.

VIII. Biliary Tumors

A. Pathogenesis
1. Carcinomas of the gallbladder and of the bile ducts are usually adenocarcinomas.
2. They are highly infiltrative and locally metastatic.
3. Both are usually associated with gallstones, although this does not establish causation.
B. Clinical and Laboratory Features
1. Carcinoma of the biliary tree is frequently not diagnosed preoperatively because of the nonspecific symptomatology, physical findings, and laboratory data. All too often, the diagnosis is discovered when jaundice has occurred or cholecystectomy is performed for another reason.
2. By the time a mass is palpable, the tumor is usually unresectable and the prognosis grave.
3. The finding of a nontender, enlarged gallbladder (Courvoisier gallbladder) may lead to the diagnosis of a cholangiocarcinoma.
4. Ampullary carcinomas may occasionally give rise to the "silver stool" comprising acholic stool mixed with occult blood.
C. Differential Diagnosis
1. Carcinoma of the gallbladder is frequently misdiagnosed as chronic cholecystitis, irritable bowel syndrome, or chronic peptic disease.

    2. Cholangiocarcinomas must be distinguished from chole-docholithiasis, postoperative or post-stone stricture, and pancreatic carcinoma.

D. Management
    1. Since these tumors are frequently diagnosed at an advanced stage, surgical resection is often not curative or feasible.
    2. These tumors tend to be resistant to chemotherapy and radiotherapy.
    3. Five-year survival of carcinomas of the gallbladder is in the range of 1–3%, and 1-year survival is less than 20%. Postoperative survival has been reported at 4–6 months.
    4. Cholangiocarcinomas may be stented surgically, via ERCP, or by transhepatic routes, but like primary cholecystic carcinomas, they have a dismal prognosis, and surgical cure is usually not possible.
    5. Two possible exceptions to this poor prognosis are:
       a. Carcinomas of the ampulla of Vater, which are more apt to create obstructive jaundice relatively early and may therefore be cured by partial gastrectomy and pancreatectomy with duodenectomy and choledochojejunostomy (Whipple procedure).
       b. Cholangiocarcinoma of the bifurcation between right and left hepatic ducts, so-called Klatskin tumor. These present with high alkaline phosphatase but little or no jaundice and may be associated with somewhat better prognosis than most cholangiocarcinomas.

IX. Postcholecystectomy Syndrome

A. Definition
    1. Catch-all term for symptoms persisting or recurring after cholecystectomy.
    2. These symptoms may be:
       a. Abdominal pain.
       b. Bloating.
       c. Eructation and/or flatulence.
       d. "Dyspepsia."
       e. Diarrhea or constipation.
       f. Abnormal "liver chemistries."

g. Jaundice.

h. Cholangitis (pain, fever, jaundice).

B. Pathogenesis

1. The original symptoms may have been attributed errone-ously to gallbladder disease, and the "postcholecystec-tomy syndrome" may represent the same illness, uninflu-enced by surgery.

2. Retained Gallstones.

a. Overlooked at the time of surgery, either too small to be seen on intraoperative cholangiogram, or pushed up into the hepatic ducts by the cholangiographic dye. About 10% of patients with cholelithiasis have coexis-tent choledocholithiasis.

b. De novo formation in ducts after cholecystectomy. This is rare, especially with pure cholesterol stones.

3. Bile Duct Stricture.

a. From previous stone passage.

b. From surgical manipulation at the time of exploration of the common bile duct.

c. From missed neoplasm of the common bile ducts.

4. "Cystic Duct Stump Syndrome."

a. Associated with large retained cystic duct.

b. May be a repository of retained stones.

c. May include a retained portion of the gallbladder.

5. "Biliary Dyskinesia." This is a complicated and somewhat controversial group of disorders involving impaired mo-tility of the bile ducts and sphincters.

C. Clinical Features and Diagnostic Studies

1. Right upper quadrant tenderness may be present, but its importance may be difficult to judge, especially in the early postoperative period.

2. Jaundice; or excoriation from itching due to deposition of bile salts in the skin.

3. Note: Common bile duct stones or strictures may not pro-duce jaundice, especially if the bile duct is not completely obstructed.

4. Laboratory tests may reveal abnormal liver markers, alka-line phosphatase, GGT, indicating biliary tract flow im-pairment. WBC may be elevated, indicative of acute infec-tion in the setting of cholangitis.

5. Ultrasonography.
   a. Will indicate common bile duct size. Duct size greater than 10 mm after cholecystectomy is generally considered abnormal.
   b. May be especially helpful for demonstrating retained stone if the common bile duct is dilated.
6. Radionuclide Scanning. May show delayed drainage from the common bile duct when obstructed but will not show stone.
7. ERCP.
   a. Will indicate duct size, strictures, stones, and cystic duct.
   b. Permits direct visualization of the duodenum and papilla.
   c. Has the potential for treatment via papillotomy and stone extraction.
8. Transhepatic Cholangiography.
   a. Like ERCP, will indicate ductular anatomy and reveal strictures, stones, and cystic duct.
   b. Most feasible when intrahepatic ducts are dilated.
   c. Does not demonstrate distal portion (bottom) of common bile duct as well as does ERCP, but is superior to ERCP in demonstrating the proximal (upper) extent of the lesion.
   d. May allow for treatment by drainage through catheters and stents.

D. Differential Diagnosis
   1. Irritable bowel syndrome.
   2. Peptic disorders (esophagitis, gastritis, duodenitis, or ulcer).
   3. Pancreatitis.
   4. Primary liver disease.
   5. Right renal colic.
   6. Diverticular disease of the colon.

E. Management
   1. Retained Stones.
      a. If detected while the T-tube (rubber tube placed intraoperatively in common bile duct and protruding through skin) is still in place postoperatively, stones can be removed by crushers and baskets or by infusion of monooctanoic acid (an emulsifying agent).

    b. ERCP: papillotomy and retrieval by crushers and baskets or other endoscopic extractors. This is successful in as many as 90% of cases in the hands of experienced endoscopists. The procedure may be complicated by bleeding, pancreatitis, perforation, or cholangitis. Antibiotics are usually administered prophylactically.

    c. Infusion of stone-dissolving substance via ERCP cannula, nasobiliary drain, transhepatic catheter, or T-tube. Solutions reported useful for this include monooctanoic acid, chenodeoxychoic acid, ursodeoxycholic acid, and ether.

    d. Repeat surgery with or without sphincteroplasty, choledochoduodenostomy, or choledochojejunostomy as Roux-en-Y.

  2. Stricture. These must be dealt with to prevent cholangitis and secondary biliary cirrhosis.

    a. ERCP with dilatation via balloon catheters or stenting.

    b. Transhepatic cholangiography with dilatation and/or stenting.

    c. Surgery.

  3. Cystic Duct Stump Syndrome. If cystic duct stump is very enlarged and contains stones, surgery is indicated.

X. Assorted "Biliary Pearls"

  A. Associated Frequency

  Approximately 10–15% of patients with cholelithiasis have coexistent choledocholithiasis.

  B. Complications

  Complications of gallstones include:

    1. Pressure necrosis of the gallbladder with fistulization to adjacent duodenum or colon (*cholecystoenteric fistula*).

    2. Migration of larger stones directly into the small intestine by fistulization, resulting in intestinal obstruction when the stone becomes lodged in the small intestine, usually in the ileum or at the site of congenital or postoperative narrowing (*gallstone ileus*).

  C. Acute Pancreatitis

  Gallstones are the major instigators of acute pancreatitis.

  D. Acalculus Cholecystitis

  Acalculus cholecystitis should be considered in patients with physical clinical pictures of cholecystitis but in whom stones cannot be detected. This is most likely to occur after burns or abdominal trauma, and in patients with collagen-vascular diseases.

XI. **Nonsurgical Eradication of Gallstones**

  A. Chenodeoxycholic Acid and Ursodeoxycholic Acid

    1. Mechanism: decrease in biliary cholesterol synthesis. Thus, bile becomes less "lithogenic."

    2. Overall efficacy: complete dissolution in 13.5% of patients with high-dose chenodeoxycholic acid (750 mg/day) for 2 years. Best results in patients with small, floating stones.

    3. Stones re-form in up to 50% of patients after therapy is stopped.

    4. Adverse side effects: increase in AST, diarrhea.

  B. Monooctanoic Acid

    1. Mechanism: emulsifying agent.

    2. Must be administered directly into biliary tree (e.g., via T-tube).

    3. Possible application: retained common duct stones after cholecystectomy and duct exploration.

  C. Lithotripsy

    Still investigational in the United States.

SUGGESTED READINGS

Schoenfield LJ, Lachin JM: Chenodiol (chenodeoxycholic acid) for dissolution of gallstones: the national cooperative gallstone study. *Ann Int Med* 95:257–282, 1984.

Thistle JF, Cleary PA, Lachin JM, et al.: The natural history of cholelithiasis: the national cooperative gallstone study. *Ann Int Med* 101:171–175, 1984.

Chapter 8

Acute Liver Disease and Hepatitis

Saul G. Agus, M.D.

VIRAL HEPATITIS

I. Introduction

Viral hepatitis is a systemic viral infection in which the particular hepatic cell necrosis gives rise to a characteristic clinical, biochemical, and morphologic pattern. There are three main varieties: hepatitis A, which is usually spread by a fecal-oral route and is self-limited; hepatitis B, which is parenterally transmitted and often becomes chronic; and non-A, non-B hepatitis, which contains many types, some of which are parenterally and some of which are fecally transmitted.

II. Approach to the Patient

A. History
1. The picture varies widely, ranging from an anicteric case with only slight malaise to a fulminant course rapidly leading to hepatic coma.
2. In the usual icteric case, there is a prodrome period, varying from days to weeks, in which the patient experiences general malaise, anorexia, nausea, perhaps flu-like symptoms with pyrexia. Shaking chills are uncommon.
3. There is generally right upper quadrant abdominal discomfort that is worsened by motion. Anorexia and malaise are

usually better in the morning. There is often loss of desire for alcohol and smoking.

4. This prodrome is usually followed by dark urine, light stool, and jaundice. There is often transient pruritus, sometimes with hives. Usually the temperature has returned to normal. Appetite may improve, but there is usually continuing lassitude and fatigue.

B. Examination

1. Depending on the stage, there may be a low-grade fever and bradycardia. Depending on the room lighting and the clinical experience of the observer, jaundice may be detectable at a bilirubin level as low as 2.0 mg/100 ml.

2. There may be transient urticaria, a few spider angiomata, scratch marks from pruritus, or other telltale cutaneous markers such as needle tracks or tattoos.

3. In 70% of cases, the liver is palpable with a smooth, tender edge. Percussion over the right lower ribs is usually uncomfortable.

4. There may be palpable splenomegaly in as many as 20% of cases.

C. Laboratory Features

Liver function tests are generally discussed in Chapter 6. As they apply particularly to viral hepatitis, however, there are several points to be noted.

1. Bilirubin will be noted in the urine before jaundice appears. There is a variable urinary threshold for bilirubin, however.

2. Urobilinogen, which is colorless, is detected in elevated amounts in the urine in the late preicteric phase. It then follows a "camel-shaped" curve, i.e., at the height of the jaundice, very little bilirubin reaches the intestine, and hence little urobilinogen is found. It reappears before final recovery and continues to be elevated until final recovery.

3. In a similar manner, the reappearance of stool color heralds impending recovery.

4. While bilirubin levels are very variable, deep jaundice implies a prolonged course.

5. Serum transaminases are very helpful in diagnosis, especially in anicteric or inapparent cases. The degree of transaminase elevation, however, is not prognostic.

6. The albumin and globulin are generally normal. The alkaline phosphatase is often elevated, but to less than three times the normal value.
7. The prothrombin time is the best prognostic guide. A prothrombin index after vitamin K administration that is less than 20% is an ominous prognostic sign.

D. Treatment

There is no specific therapy for acute hepatitis. Early diagnosis and notification of individuals at risk may have some preventive value.

1. Rest is important, although it need not be bed-rest. A low-fat, high-carbohydrate diet is more palatable to an anorectic patient. High-quality proteins are important in the recovery phase.
2. Corticosteroids are generally not indicated except for patients with prolonged cholestasis.

III. Hepatitis A

A. Characteristics of the Virus

1. Hepatitis A is caused by a 27-nm cubically symmetric RNA picornavirus. It has been identified in the stools of individuals with acute hepatitis A for a period of about 2 weeks prior to and 1 week after the onset of jaundice.
2. The virus has been grown in tissue culture and has been transmitted to chimpanzees.
3. It seems to be directly cytopathic.

B. Epidemiology

1. Hepatitis A is generally spread by the fecal/oral route. It has an incubation period of 15–50 days. In rare cases, it can be transmitted by transfusion of infected blood.
2. The highest incidence is in children between ages 5 and 14 years. Adults often become infected from children.
3. There have been several food-borne and water-borne epidemics. In addition, there have been several epidemics following the ingestion of raw clams and oysters from contaminated waters. Steaming is often inadequate.

C. Clinical Course

1. In children, the disease is often mild, and is passed off as gastroenteritis. Adults tend to be sicker.

2. There are occasional cases of fulminant hepatitis that may be due to a high dose of virus or impaired immune responses.
3. The mortality rate is approximately 0.1%.
4. Chronicity or a chronic carrier state does not develop.

D. Laboratory Tests
1. Antibody to the hepatitis A virus (anti-HAV) appears in the serum as the stool becomes negative. It reaches a maximum in several months but is detectable for many years. This antibody may be protective against further attack.
2. Serum immunoglobulin M (IgM) anti-HAV persists for only 2–6 months and is hence more specific for acute infection.
3. A liver biopsy would show typical hepatic cell necrosis with leukocytic and histocytic reaction. There may be cellular infiltration of the portal zone and evidence of cholestasis.

E. Prevention
1. Hepatitis A is difficult to control, since most of its fecal shedding occurs before the clinical illness.
2. Conscientious hand-washing is important, as is the implementation of strict general hygienic practices.
3. Immune serum globulin is helpful if it is given early enough. Generally, 3 ml given within 10 days of exposure is prophylactic.
4. There is no widely accepted vaccine at present.

IV. Hepatitis B (HB)

A. Characteristics of the Virus
1. Hepatitis B virus (HBV) is one of the hepadnaviruses. It is a small, double-shelled spherical virus. The nucleocapsid is an icosahedron 27 nm in diameter, surrounded by a detergent-sensitive, lipid-rich envelope 42 nm in diameter.
2. The lipid of the envelope is derived from the host. In addition, the envelope contains at least three polypeptides. The major protein, 226 amino acids long, corresponds to hepatitis B surface antigen (HBsAg).
3. Hepadnaviruses have partially double-stranded and partially single-stranded circular DNA. Replication resembles that of a retrovirus in that it involves a reverse transcriptase.

    4. Hepatitis B core antigen (HBcAg) is the major antigenic protein of the HBV nucleocapsid.

    5. e-Antigen (HBeAg) is a degradation product of the HBcAg. The presence of HBeAg in the serum is indicative of a replicative phase of the virus.

    6. HBsAg particles have antigenically complex surfaces. These subtypes breed true and are helpful in tracing the course of epidemics. They apparently have no clinical significance.

B. Epidemiology

    1. Hepatitis B usually is spread by whole blood and its products. Semen and saliva are also probably infectious. Transmission is parenteral or by intimate contact.

    2. The carrier rate for hepatitis B surface antigen varies from 0.1% in the United States to about 15% in Hong Kong. There are thus millions of carriers in the world.

    3. The majority of carriers seem to be healthy. Some suffer from chronic hepatitis, and some develop cirrhosis and liver cancer.

    4. Vertical transmission from mother to neonate may be an important mode of spread.

    5. There are other reservoirs of chronic HBV infection, including drug abusers, prostitutes, homosexuals, paid blood donors, staff and patients of hospitals for the mentally retarded, and renal dialysis patients.

    6. Mosquitoes and bedbugs play an unknown role. The virus seems not to replicate in them, but rather to be passively excreted.

C. Clinical Course

    1. Subclinical episodes are common.

    2. The usual clinical attack is similar to what was described for HAV, although sometimes more severe.

    3. In addition to the usual features of hepatitis, there may be a "serum sickness-like" syndrome suggesting immune complex disease. This is characterized by fever, urticaria, and arthropathy. Serum complement levels are often reduced.

    4. There are several extrahepatic immune complex-related diseases in which HBsAg plays a role. Among these are several cases of polyarteritis, glomerulonephritis, polymyal-

gia rheumatica, mixed cryoglobulinemia, Guillain-Barré syndrome, and myocarditis.

5. Exposure to HBV has results ranging from no clinical attack in some to a fulminant attack in others. In general, the more acute and the more severe attacks are associated with a lower incidence of chronic disease.
6. Immunocompromised individuals are more likely to develop chronicity.

D. Serology of HBV
1. HBsAg usually appears days to weeks after exposure but before the transaminase elevation. HBsAg persists for a few weeks to several months after the icteric phase.
2. HBeAg usually appears a few days after HBsAg but is often transient. When HBeAg disappears, the corresponding antibody, anti-HBe, usually appears.
3. The first antibody to appear is usually against the core antigen (anti-HBc). Initially, this is both IgM and immunoglobulin G (IgG). In 4–6 months, the IgM titer falls and IgG anti-HBc becomes predominant.
4. After HBsAg disappears, anti-HBs becomes detectable, usually in the recovery phase.

E. Hepatitis B Carrier State
1. About 10% of patients contracting hepatitis B will not clear HBsAg from the serum within 6 months.
2. Hepatitis B carriers may show changes on liver biopsy even in the presence of normal blood tests. These changes may vary from persistent hepatitis to chronic hepatitis with cirrhosis.
3. It has been estimated that there may be a worldwide reservoir of as many as 300 million hepatitis carriers.
4. After a long period of latency, there is, in addition, an increased risk of hepatocellular carcinoma in these carriers.

F. Prevention
1. Hepatitis B immune globulin (HBIG) is effective for passive immunization against hepatitis B if given prophylactically or within hours of infection.
2. It is indicated for victims of parenteral exposure to HBsAg-positive blood, sexual contacts of individuals with acute hepatitis B, and neonates born to HBsAg-positive mothers.
3. In addition to HBIG, hepatitis B vaccine should be initiated as well.

4. Hepatitis B vaccine is strongly suggested for health care workers in contact with hepatitis B patients, sexual contacts of HBV carriers, homosexuals, babies born to HBsAg-positive mothers, drug abusers, and children in institutions for the mentally retarded.

5. The first vaccine available was Heptavax-B, which was prepared from plasma of hepatitis B carriers. The vaccine has been shown to be safe and effective. There is also Recombivax-HB available, which is synthetically prepared by recombinant-DNA technology. Since it is free of plasma, it has had wider acceptability.

V. Delta Hepatitis (HD)

A. Viral Characteristics
   1. Hepatitis delta virus (HDV) is 35–37 nm in diameter. The core bears the antigenic protein (HDVAg), and the envelope incorporates HBsAg.
   2. The genome is a single-stranded circular RNA. It depends upon the DNA genome of HBV for its maturation, although its RNA shares no homology with HB DNA.

B. Epidemiology
   1. HDV occurs only in HBsAg-positive individuals. It is highly infectious.
   2. It has been reported in endemic form in Italy, in the Mediterranean basin, and in the Third World. In addition, it is now being found in intravenous drug abusers, hemophiliacs, and male homosexuals throughout the world.

C. Clinical Course
   1. The incubation period is from 2 to 12 weeks. The clinical picture depends on whether there is simultaneous coinfection or subsequent superinfection of a chronic HB carrier with δ agent.
   2. Coinfection with HBV and HDV is almost indistinguishable from acute HB except that the disease is often more fulminant. Often, there is a biphasic or relapsing hepatitis, but the δ agent cannot outlive the HBs antigenemia.
   3. δ Agent superinfection should always be considered in any hepatitis B carrier who has a relapse.
   4. Although the synthesis of hepatitis B viral particles is reduced in the presence of δ virus, the resultant chronic hepatitis is accelerated.

D. Serology
1. Low or rising anti-HDV titers are found during the acute phase of HDV, whereas chronic HDV is associated with a high titer of antibody.
2. In addition, IgM-specific anti-HDV is more specific for acute HDV infection. Resolution of HDV infection is followed by disappearance of the IgM-specific anti-HDV antibody.
E. Prevention
1. Hepatitis B vaccine, by preventing hepatitis B infection, will also prevent HDV infection.
2. This is particularly important because HBsAg carriers with persistent HDV infection may be at increased risk for hepatoma.

VI. **Non-A, Non-B Hepatitis (NANB)**

A. Virology
1. There are at least two different viral agents with different modes of spread for non-A, non-B hepatitis.
2. The first is posttransfusion NANB hepatitis, which is epidemiologically similar to hepatitis B. This is the most common NANB hepatitis in North America.
3. The second type is enterically transmitted (ET-NANB). Large outbreaks of ET-NANB hepatitis have occurred in Africa, Asia, the Soviet Union, and Mexico.
B. Diagnosis
1. The diagnosis of NANB hepatitis depends on the exclusion of other known forms of hepatitis, such as HA, HB, cytomegalovirus (CMV), and Epstein-Barr virus.
2. With ET-NANB, 28- to 34-nm virus-like particles have been found in the stool and sera of acutely ill patients.
C. Clinical
1. NANB hepatitis accounts for about 97% of posttransfusion jaundice.
2. There is a high incidence of chronic hepatitis and cirrhosis, often without symptoms.
3. ET-NANB carries a high mortality, especially in pregnant women.
D. Prevention and Treatment

1. Since the antigens and antibodies of NANB hepatitis have only very recently been isolated, specific tests for their presence are not yet generally available, but they probably will be within a few years.
2. In the absence of specific tests, screening of blood for transaminase elevation and for anti-HBc can reduce the incidence of posttransfusion hepatitis.
3. There is no specific therapy for NANB hepatitis. γ-Globulin is of no proven merit. Corticosteroids are of little benefit.

VII. **Other Infectious Causes of Hepatitis**

  A. Infectious Mononucleosis
    1. Infectious mononucleosis is caused by the Epstein-Barr virus and may mimic NANB hepatitis. There may be fever, abdominal discomfort without the pharyngitis, lymphadenopathy, and splenomegaly with an acute attack.
    2. Overt jaundice is unusual. The serum transaminases and alkaline phosphatase may be elevated.
    3. Pathologically, there is often a diffuse mononuclear infiltration of the liver.
    4. IgM antibodies to EBV antigens will give a specific diagnosis.
  B. Cytomegalovirus (CMV)
    1. CMV hepatitis is an important cause of posttransfusion hepatitis. It may simulate HBV, HAV, or NANB hepatitis.
    2. Sometimes it is characterized by fever that continues after the onset of jaundice, which is not common with other forms of hepatitis.
    3. Histologically, one may find noncaseating granulomas or cholestasis.
    4. In immunosuppressed patients, there may be a generalized CMV infection, which can be fatal.
  C. Other Viruses
    1. Among common viruses, hepatitis may be caused by measles, varicella, coxsackievirus B, adenovirus, and herpes simplex.
    2. There are several newly discovered, highly dangerous viral illnesses in which the liver may be involved. In this group are Ebola virus, Marburg virus, and Lassa fever.

VIII. The Liver in AIDS

A. Neoplasms
1. The most common tumor in AIDS patients is Kaposi's sarcoma (KS).
2. When KS involves the liver, usually other organs such as the bowel or lungs are involved as well.
3. Lymphomas, especially non-Hodgkin's type, are common in AIDS patients and may be detected in the liver in primary or metastatic form.
B. Infectious Diseases in the Liver of AIDS Patients
1. Hepatitis B is the most common viral disease affecting the liver in AIDS patients. While some patients with AIDS and chronic hepatitis tend to have a mild course, some have a progressive course leading to chronic active hepatitis and cirrhosis.
2. NANB hepatitis is found in AIDS patients, but its frequency does not seem to differ from its occurrence in other high-risk groups.
3. Evidence of HAV infection is common in AIDS patients. The behavior of this virus in AIDS patients is unknown.
4. CMV may involve the liver in up to 44% of AIDS cases, primarily by dissemination from the lung. It may also involve the biliary tract in unusual ways.
5. Mycobacterial infection is not uncommon in AIDS. Clinically, this is usually manifested as fever, hepatomegaly, and an elevated alkaline phosphatase. The liver may be the only site of involvement. Among Haitians with AIDS, *Mycobacterium tuberculosis* is the most common organism. Among non-Haitians, *M. avium* and *M. intracellulare* are the most common.
6. *Cryptococcus neoformans* is the most common fungal infection in AIDS patients. Histoplasmosis, candidiasis, and toxoplasmosis have also been found in AIDS patients.

CHRONIC HEPATITIS

I. Introduction

Chronic inflammation of the liver continuing at least 6 months constitutes chronic hepatitis. (See also Chapter 9.) Chronic hepatitis is generally subdivided into chronic persistent hepatitis, chronic lobular hepatitis, and chronic active hepatitis. The histologic distinctions go far beyond the scope of this book. However, in general terms, chronic hepatitis implies the possibility of reversibility; i.e., the zonal architecture of the liver is preserved. In cirrhosis, on the other hand, there is an irreversible change in the hepatic architecture, with the development of fibrosis and nodular regeneration. Classification based on histology is of some importance in that chronic persistent and chronic lobular hepatitis do not progress to cirrhosis.

II. Chronic Persistent Hepatitis (CPH)

A. Etiology and Clinical Features
1. The cause of chronic persistent hepatitis (CPH) is usually unknown. The patient may have no symptoms or very vague symptoms.
2. Biochemical parameters are usually not strikingly elevated. The serum γ-globulin level is usually normal.

B. Liver biopsy
1. This is the only definitive way to distinguish CPH from chronic active hepatitis.
2. The biopsy will also help to exclude Gilbert's syndrome and alcoholic liver disease.

C. Treatment and Prognosis
1. There is no specific treatment.
2. The prognosis is excellent. Those patients who are HBsAg and e-antigen positive are a little more refractory.

III. Chronic Lobular Hepatitis (CLH)

This is a rare condition that is diagnosed by liver biopsy. There are a variety of possible causes. The important feature is that there is an excellent response to prednisolone therapy and cirrhosis does not develop.

IV. Chronic Active Hepatitis (CAH)

A. Etiology
There are several diverse etiologies that can lead to the clinical and pathologic picture of chronic active hepatitis. Since the treatments

for the diverse conditions may well be different, it is important to perform certain tests and to get appropriate historical background to make the differentiation.

1. Alcohol-related disease is discussed in Chapter 9.
2. Wilson's disease is discussed in Chapter 9.
3. α-1-Antitrypsin deficiency is discussed in Chapter 9.
4. Rubella and CMV are unusual.
5. Drug-induced hepatitis, especially due to methyldopa, isoniazid, nitrofurantoin, dantrolene, and laxatives containing oxyphenisatine. The treatment is discontinuation of the offending drug.
6. Chronic active hepatitis B. In the progressive form, this disease responds poorly to steroids and progresses to cirrhosis, portal hypertension, and death.
7. Chronic active non-A, non-B hepatitis.
8. Chronic active hepatitis with immunologic features. This condition occurs primarily in females and is characterized by hyperglobulinemia, a positive antinuclear antibody, and often a positive lupus erythematosus (LE) prep. Clinically, there is often fatigue, fever, rash, arthritis, and amenorrhea.

B. Treatment
1. The patients described above with CAH and immunologic features will often respond to therapy with prednisolone with or without azathioprine. Long-term therapy is the rule, as premature cessation of therapy leads to relapse.
2. Long-term trials of prednisolone therapy for patients with CAH at the Mayo Clinic and at the Royal Free Hospital have shown enhanced survival in the corticosteroid-treated group, although most patients did eventually become cirrhotic.
3. Patients who are HBsAg-positive and have chronic active hepatitis are a problem. There are some data that suggest that we should identify those individuals who have evidence of active viral replication, i.e., HBeAg+, anti-HBe−, HBV DNA+. In these individuals, antiviral therapy may have something to offer. On the other hand, in those individuals in whom the HB-viral genome has already incorporated itself into the host's genome, immunosuppressive therapy may be more appropriate. Such individuals are usually HBcAg−, anti-HBe+, and HBV DNA−.

4. Another promising area of therapeutic research involves d-interferon, which is discussed further in Chapter 9.

DRUGS AND THE LIVER

I. **Introduction**

We are surrounded by chemicals in the modern world. Many chemical agents can produce hepatic injury. Some drugs are toxic intrinsically, some as a result of an idiosyncratic reaction in the individual. Some drugs are directly cytotoxic. Some produce arrested bile flow and jaundice (cholestasis). In addition, in the present world, there is concern about the chronic effects of certain drugs and their ability to cause chronic liver disease and neoplasia.

II. **Intrinsic Hepatotoxins**

A. Direct Hepatotoxins
   1. These agents are capable of injuring the liver by a direct physicochemical effect.
   2. Histologically, there is necrosis and steatosis.
   3. Chemicals in this category include CCl_4, $CHCl_3$, and phosphorus.

B. Indirect Hepatotoxins
   1. These are generally antimetabolites that interfere with a specific metabolic pathway, which then leads to a structural injury.
   2. Cytotoxic indirect hepatotoxins lead to steatosis, necrosis, or combinations of both. In this group are antibiotics and antimetabolites used in therapy, such as tetracycline, L-asparaginase, methotrexate, 6-mercaptopurine, and plicamycin.
   3. Ethanol is an indirect hepatotoxin that leads to necrosis as well as fatty metamorphosis. (See Chapter 9).
   4. Cholestatic indirect hepatotoxins selectively interfere with the biliary excretion system and lead to jaundice. In this category are anabolic steroids, oral contraceptives, and estradiol.

C. Idiosyncratic Hepatic Injury
   1. Hypersensitivity-related reactions tend to involve fever, rash, and eosinophilia.

2. These reactions are not dose-dependent.
3. The incidence is low.
4. Some drugs that have been associated with hypersensitivity-related reactions are halothane, chlorpromazine, oral hypoglycemic agents, and isoniazid. In some of these cases, there is metabolic derangement as well.

D. Drugs Implicated in Chronic Active Hepatitis
   1. A number of drugs have been implicated in producing an inflammatory lesion that resembles CAH (see "Chronic Hepatitis").
   2. Included in this list are oxyphenisatine, methyldopa, isoniazid, nitrofurantoin, dantrolene, sulfonamides, propylthiouracil, and chlorpromazine. Methotrexate leads to portal fibrosis.

E. Drugs and Hepatic Tumors
   1. Oral contraceptives in particular have been associated with hepatic adenomas as well as with peliosis hepatis.
   2. Thorotrast has led to hepatoma, cholangiocarcinoma, and angiosarcoma.
   3. Angiosarcoma has been associated with exposure to vinyl chloride.

III. Drug Challenge

There are many times when one suspects a certain drug in causing mild hepatic abnormalities. In some cases, challenge with small doses of the drug may be the only way to ascertain the toxicity. This is fraught with a lot of potential risk and is not to be undertaken lightly. This challenge may be accompanied by a liver biopsy to further assess the mechanism of the hepato-toxicity.

FULMINANT HEPATIC FAILURE

I. Overview

This syndrome of massive hepatic necrosis occurring within the context of acute liver disease progresses rapidly to liver failure and coma. The mortality is high, with survival approximately 15–30% despite maximal therapy. Young age is a relatively better prognostic factor. The pathogenesis is unclear, although host factors are felt to be important.

II. Etiology

Etiologies include viral hepatitis (worst in non-A, non-B, but occurring also in hepatitis B, delta hepatitis, and hepatitis A); drugs and toxins (especially acetaminophen); Wilson's disease; fatty liver of pregnancy; and Reye's syndrome. In the latter two epidemiologies, microvesicular fat is the histologic hallmark.

III. Clinical Manifestations

Clinically, fulminant hepatic failure (FHF) presents as altered mental status usually (but not always) in a patient recognized to have hepatitis, which progresses rapidly to coma. Patients are deeply jaundiced. A shrinking liver is a poor sign. The prothrombin time is markedly abnormal, and there may be low-grade disseminated intravascular coagulation (DIC). Half the patients bleed from the gastrointestinal tract. Respiratory failure, hypoglycemia, renal failure, and adult respiratory distress syndrome (ARDS) may be noted. Patients often develop secondary bacterial infections. Laboratory findings include bilirubin levels as high as 40 mg/dl and aminotransferases typical for viral hepatitis. Aminotransferases may seem to "normalize" terminally. The serum α-fetoprotein may be elevated, implying regeneration.

IV. Treatment

To a large extent, treatment is aimed at supporting the patient until his/her own liver regenerates. Treatment includes: endotracheal intubation if required, antibiotics if required for a specific infection, lactulose (by enema if necessary), and vitamin K. Serum glucose should be monitored frequently and hypoglycemia treated with intravenous 10% or 20% dextrose solutions (D10 or D20). Histamine-2 (H-2) receptor antagonists may be used. In the past, many measures were tried, including corticosteroid usage, charcoal hemoperfusion, hemodialysis, exchange transfusions, and extracorporeal hepatic perfusion. None was found to significantly affect mortality. Liver transplantation has been successfully attempted in patients with FHF and should be strongly considered. Patients who survive FHF secondary to viral hepatitis eventually regenerate their liver with normal architecture. They do not manifest chronic hepatitis.

SUGGESTED READING

Van Thiel DH: Viral hepatitis. *Gastroenterol Forum* 1:2–15, 1988.

Chapter 9

Chronic Liver Disease and Cirrhosis

Barbara Kapelman, M.D.

I. General Considerations

  A. Introduction

    The term "chronic liver disease" encompasses a broad range of hepatic abnormalities, from mild increases in enzyme activities of little clinical significance to cirrhosis, with its attendant complications and mortality. Cirrhosis itself is the end stage of a variety of hepatic disease processes. Properly speaking, the diagnosis is made on histologic grounds (see below). In practice, however, clinical considerations including abnormal clotting parameters may preclude a liver biopsy, and a "working diagnosis" must be arrived at on clinical grounds.

  B. Clinical Presentation

    1. Physical Findings. Signs of portal hypertension and liver failure are highly suggestive of chronic liver disease and cirrhosis. Occasionally, they may be secondary to non-hepatic causes or to acute liver disease. Occasionally they may be absent. Signs include: ascites, esophageal varices, hepatosplenomegaly (or liver may be shrunken), spider angiomata, palmar erythema, caput medusae, gynecomastia, clubbing, Terry's nails, Muercke's lines, asterixis, and signs of deeper encephalopathy, including coma.

    2. Laboratory Findings. Standard liver tests cannot distin-

guish acute from chronic disease or chronic noncirrhotic disease from cirrhosis. Occasionally, liver test results may be normal. Certain laboratory findings may be suggestive but not diagnostic of chronic liver disease with cirrhosis. These include: pancytopenia (suggestive of hypersplenism secondary to portal hypertension); anemia (macrocytic secondary to alcohol use or folate deficiency, microcytic secondary to chronic blood loss); hypoalbuminemia (implying chronic rather than acute disease); elevated prothrombin time (more likely to be chronic, but if present acutely may signify fulminant hepatic failure, or may be secondary to cholestasis); hyponatremia; target cells; β-γ bridging on serum protein electrophoresis (SPEP); elevated ammonia level (an imperfect test, see section on ammonia below).

3. Child-Turcotte Classification. In 1964, Child and Turcotte published a classification for use in patients with cirrhosis. It is shown in Table 9.1.

Classification is simple when all five criteria for a given patient fall into the same category. It is trickier when they do not, especially since there is no standard for scoring the different groups. Nonetheless, the concept of classification is important and useful in assessing severity and prognosis in chronic liver disease.

Table 9.1.
Criteria for Child-Turcotte Classification[a]

Group designation	A	B	C
Serum bilirubin (mg/100 ml)	Below 2.0	2.0–3.0	Over 3.0
Serum albumin (g/100 ml)	Over 3.5	3.0–3.5	Under 3.0
Ascites	None	Easily controlled	Poorly controlled
Neurological disorder	None	Minimal	Advanced "coma"
Nutrition	Excellent	Good	Poor, "wasting"

[a]From Conn HO: A peek at the Child-Turcotte classification. *Hepatology* 1:674, 1981.

C. Histology
1. General Considerations.
    a. Chronic persistent hepatitis, chronic active hepatitis, and cirrhosis are conditions whose diagnoses are based on *histology*, although the terms are often used as if they can be identified on clinical grounds. In a given patient, histology, symptoms, and results of liver tests may not correlate well with each other.
    b. The small size of a percutaneous liver biopsy specimen (estimated at 1/100,000 of the liver volume) allows for possible sampling error. This is less likely in diffuse diseases such as acute viral hepatitis and relatively more likely in focal conditions such as metastatic disease.
2. Cirrhosis. Cirrhosis is defined histologically as the presence of nodules of hepatocytic parenchyma surrounded by a 360° rim of collagen, with distortion of liver architecture. The degree of active inflammation and ongoing lobular destruction varies greatly. The nodules may be regenerative or may be formed by collapse and fibrosis. The size of the nodules varies from less than 3 mm (micronodular) to many centimeters (macronodular). Nodules larger than the diameter of the biopsy needle can produce a specimen that does not show the rim of collagen despite true cirrhosis. Also, a cirrhotic specimen may fragment, confounding the diagnosis. Occasionally, the needle may sample only a regenerating nodule, resulting in a relatively normal specimen.
D. Treatment
The treatment of cirrhosis involves the treatment of its complications, to a large extent. These are discussed below. Where specific therapy exists for a given condition, it will be covered in the discussion of that condition.

Medical therapy for cirrhosis has received attention recently. Colchicine may improve mortality in patients with cirrhosis secondary to a number of etiologies, especially alcohol abuse (1).

The advent of liver transplantation has meant hope for many patients with chronic liver disease. Refinements in technique and immunosuppression have improved 1-year survival to approximately 80%. Timing of the procedure is important. Remaining life span and quality of life must be assessed versus surgical mortality. After the acute period, postoperative quality of life is quite good. If the operation is performed too late in the course of disease, surgical mortality increases.

II. Causes of Chronic Liver Disease

A. Infectious Causes of Chronic Liver Disease
1. Chronic Viral Hepatitis.
   a. Hepatitis A does not cause chronic liver disease.
   b. Hepatitis B. Morbidity and mortality secondary to chronic hepatitis B (including hepatocellular carcinoma) are major problems worldwide. Carrier rates vary from 0.1–0.5% in the United States to 5% around the Mediterranean to approximately 20% in the Far East. There is also a significant incidence in sub-Saharan Africa. In the latter areas, maternal-neonatal transmission is significant.

   Patients becoming icteric from acute hepatitis represent only a small fraction of people infected. The diagnosis of hepatitis B is often made in retrospect when the patient presents with sequelae of chronic hepatitis or cirrhosis. Five percent of people infected acquire chronic hepatitis; 20–25% of these become cirrhotic. Usually surface antigen is present, although on occasion only the surface and core antibodies or core antibody alone may implicate hepatitis B. The definition of chronicity varies. Many centers accept 6 months of abnormal aminotransferase activity with persistent surface antigen. We prefer a criterion of 1 year, since liver biopsy before this time can confuse chronic hepatitis with resolving acute hepatitis. Spontaneous conversion from the surface antigen-positive state to the negative state occurs at a rate of approximately 1% of patients per year. Spontaneous conversion from the e antigen-positive state to the negative state occurs at a rate of approximately 8–12% per year.

   Patients who are hepatitis B surface antigen-positive should be counselled concerning transmission of disease via sexual contact, blood, and blood products, regardless of their histologic category. Sexual contacts of these patients are candidates for the hepatitis B vaccine. Neonates born to hepatitis B surface antigen-positive mothers should receive hyperimmune globulin as well as the vaccine soon after delivery. This decreases the likelihood that the child will develop chronic hepatitis B.

i. Asymptomatic Chronic Carriers: Some patients present with surface antigen in the blood (with or without e antigen) yet have normal results of liver tests and are asymptomatic. Liver biopsy is not necessary unless the patient is to enter into a research study. If e antigen is present, check it every 6–12 months until it becomes negative, then check the surface antigen every 6–12 months. α-Fetoprotein (AFP) should be monitored periodically, especially in long-standing carriers.

ii. Chronic Persistent Hepatitis. Signs and symptoms are often absent. Some patients complain of fatigue, anorexia, depression, and sleep disorders. Mild hepatomegaly may be noted. Histologically there is infiltration of portal tracts by lymphocytes and plasma cells with maintenance of the limiting plate. Fibrosis is minimal if present at all. There may be scattered areas of focal necrosis in the parenchyma, whose architecture is otherwise maintained. "Ground glass" cells have a frosted pink appearance on hematoxylin and eosin (H&E) stain and represent endoplasmic reticulum forming excess surface antigen. This condition usually does not progress to cirrhosis. Hepatitis B surface and e antigens and AFP should be monitored as for the asymptomatic carrier state. Follow results of liver tests as well.

iii. Chronic Active Hepatitis. Symptoms include fatigue, anorexia, depression, and sleep problems. Some patients are asymptomatic. Hepato(spleno)megaly may be noted. Extrahepatic manifestations include rash, arthritis, polyarteritis, and glomerulonephritis. Aminotransferase activities range from near normal to approximately 700 units. The alkaline phosphatase activity may be normal to several times normal. Jaundice depends on the severity of disease. Symptoms and liver tests may fluctuate in recurrent bouts of disease. As the disease progresses, complications of cirrhosis may develop. Hepatocellular carcinoma (HCC) may supervene.

Histologically, chronic active hepatitis is defined as the presence of (a) piecemeal necrosis, i.e., lymphocytes and plasma cells extending past the limiting plate and engulfing one or several hepatocytes in a piecemeal fashion; and (b) bridging necrosis consisting of bands of connective tissue extending from portal to portal areas and, more important, from portal to centrilobular areas.

At present, there is no accepted treatment for chronic hepatitis secondary to the hepatitis B virus. Extensive research is underway using a variety of agents, most notably α-interferon. The objects are to reduce serum levels of hepatitis B virus deoxyribonucleic acid (HBV DNA) and deoxyribonucleic acid (DNA) polymerase and to convert HBeAg-positive patients to the HBeAg-negative state. There is evidence of efficacy in some patients (2). Corticosteroids are contraindicated in surface antigen-positive patients. Monitor liver test results and α-fetoprotein.

iv. Hepatitis D (Delta). This condition is a subset of hepatitis B, since the incomplete hepatitis D virus requires surface antigen as its outer coat. Therefore, only patients who are hepatitis B surface antigen-positive are at risk for delta infection. It may be acquired simultaneously with hepatitis B ("coinfection") or as a subsequent infection ("superinfection"). It must be strongly considered in surface antigen-positive patients with sudden deterioration. Patients with delta hepatitis have more severe disease than those without it.

c. Non-A, Non-B Hepatitis. Chronic hepatitis secondary to (one of) the non-A, non-B virus(es) is a significant problem in patients who have received multiple transfusions. Although most patients seem to have mild disease, there is a higher percentage of chronicity (>50%) than with hepatitis B. The diagnosis, as for acute non-A, non-B hepatitis, currently is one of exclusion. A serologic test may become available soon. Epstein-Barr virus (EBV) and cytomegalovirus (CMV) must be ruled out.

Marked fluctuations in aminotransferase activities may occur. On liver biopsy, bile duct damage and fatty change are prominent, unlike in hepatitis B. There is no accepted treatment, although research is being conducted using the same agents used for hepatitis B.

2. Schistosomiasis. Schistosomiasis (bilharziasis) is an infection by trematode worms acquired by wading through contaminated water in Puerto Rico, Egypt, South America, Africa, and the Far East. Three species, *Schistosoma haematobium* (terminal spine), *S. japonicum* (vestigial spine), and *S. mansoni* (lateral spine), are important, the latter two causing hepatic disease. Eggs lodge in the small intrahepatic portal veins and cause granuloma formation. On cut liver section, the large areas of portal fibrosis produced a characteristic appearance likened to a clay "pipe-stem" cut crosswise. The ensuing portal hypertension is "pre-sinusoidal" with normal intrahepatic pressure. Bleeding secondary to esophageal varices is a common presentation. Hepatosplenomegaly is present, but other sequelae of chronic liver disease are not pronounced, since the hepatic parenchyma functions fairly well. The alkaline phosphatase activity is frequently mildly elevated, but the aminotransferase activity and bilirubin are usually normal. The diagnosis is made by finding eggs in the stool, or on rectal or liver biopsy. Since hepatic disease may present 10–15 years after initial infection, stool specimens may be negative because of intercurrent treatment or death of egg-laying adults. Radioimmunoassay and enzyme-linked immunosorbent assay (ELISA) are sensitive blood tests but do not distinguish current from prior infection. Treatment of schistosomiasis is oral praziquantel. While this treats active infection, well-established portal hypertension and its sequelae must be managed in the usual fashion.

3. Echinococcosis (Hydatidosis). Echinococcosis (hydatidosis) is a cestode (tapeworm) infection caused by *Echinococcus* species. The most common is the "pastoral" form of *E. granulosis*, which causes cysts in the liver and lungs. It is spread by dogs, especially in sheep-raising countries, i.e., Greece, Uruguay, Argentina, the Middle East, Australia, and New Zealand. The "sylvatic" form, present in Alaska and western Canada, is more benign. Many patients are asymptomatic, but large cysts can cause abdominal pain and

a palpable mass. A calcified cystic lesion on x-ray is suggestive of the diagnosis. Twenty-five percent of patients have eosinophilia. There may be a latent period of many years; therefore, the condition should be considered in a patient migrating from an endemic area. Complications include rupture into the biliary tree, peritoneum, pleural cavity, or bronchus. Fever, urticaria, and fatal anaphylaxis may ensue. *E. multilocularis* causes an alveolar hydatid disease that presents as a slowly growing tumor.

Treatment of echinococcosis is surgical. During excision, care should be taken not to spill the contents into the abdominal cavity. Medical therapy with mebendazole or related compounds is used only in patients who are not surgical candidates. Often treatment is not necessary.

B. Drugs and Toxins That Cause Chronic Liver Disease

1. Alcohol. The ingestion of ethyl alcohol (ethanol, alcohol) in significant quantities leads to four types of liver injury: fatty liver, alcoholic hepatitis, cirrhosis, and, indirectly, hepatocellular carcinoma. The definition of "significant intake" varies based on individual susceptibility, which is poorly understood. As a general rule, ingestion of 80 grams of alcohol per day for 15 years will cause liver disease. This equates with more than 8 cans of beer, a liter of wine, or half a pint of 80 proof whiskey per day. Each of the four entities will be discussed in turn.

a. Fatty Liver. Alcohol is one of several causes of a fatty liver. (For a general discussion of fatty liver, see II.C.1.) Alcohol acts in several ways to derange lipid metabolism and cause the build-up of excess triglyceride in the liver. Alcoholic fatty liver is suggested in a patient with a large, smooth liver and recent or prolonged alcohol usage. Tenderness may or may not be present. In uncomplicated fatty liver, signs of hepatic decompensation are infrequent. Jaundice is present in one-quarter of cases. The aspartate aminotransferase (AST) is usually less than 300 units/L. The alkaline phosphatase activity may be normal or moderately elevated. The white blood count is usually normal. Uncomplicated fatty liver can resolve completely and generally is not felt to cause cirrhosis, although there is discussion on this point. Sometimes a fatty liver may be seen in conjunction with alcoholic hepatitis. In this case, the syndrome produced is more characteristic of the alcoholic hepatitis (see below). The treatment of an alcoholic fatty liver is abstention and supportive care.

b. Alcoholic Hepatitis. Alcoholic hepatitis is a syndrome of liver damage which is characterized histologically by ballooning degeneration and necrosis of hepatocytes, and infiltration with polymorphonuclear leukocytes. The damaged hepatocytes may contain Mallory bodies (alcoholic hyalin), which stain as purple-red clumps with H&E stain. This material represents intermediate filaments (cytokeratin) that are normally part of the hepatocyte cytoskeleton. Mallory bodies are not pathognomonic for alcohol toxicity but may be seen in fatty liver secondary to other causes, as well as in primary biliary cirrhosis, hepatocellular carcinoma, and Wilson's disease. Fat may be present to a variable degree. Fibrosis is often present and varies from fine fibrils surrounding individual hepatocytes to frank cirrhosis. This latter syndrome of active necrosis and inflammation complicating cirrhosis is sometimes called florid cirrhosis. Multiple terms are used to denote fibrosis around terminal hepatitis venules (central veins), e.g., *perivenular sclerosis, central hyalin sclerosis,* and *sclerosing hyalin necrosis.* This lesion may progress to cirrhosis. Evidence of cholestasis and of iron overload (usually in Kupffer cells) may be noted as well.

Clinically, alcoholic hepatitis is characterized by fatigue, anorexia, nausea, vomiting, and a large tender liver. Jaundice (sometimes prolonged), fever, and a leukocytosis are often noted. Stigmata of chronic liver disease are common but not invariable. Evidence of protein-calorie malnutrition is common. The AST is abnormal in most patients but is usually less than 200–300 units/L. Unlike viral hepatitis, the AST is higher than the alanine aminotransferase (ALT). The alkaline phosphatase activity is usually elevated, but not more than about twice normal. The γ-glutamyl transpeptidase activity may be dramatically elevated (600 units/L or greater). However, it is not a good measure of the degree of liver injury, since it is subject to microsomal enzyme induction by alcohol. On occasion, alcoholic hepatitis may exhibit marked cholestasis, with bilirubin values of 18 mg/dl or greater. This syndrome of cholestatic alcoholic hepatitis must be distinguished from true mechanical biliary obstruction, since surgery on these patients carries a high mortality. Other laboratory abnormalities include an elevated prothrombin time, low serum albumin, and anemia with a high mean corpuscular volume (MCV).

Patients with alcoholic hepatitis often get worse after hospital admission despite abstention from alcohol, good nutrition, and supportive care. The condition carries an acute mortality ranging from 17 to 44% depending on severity of disease on presentation. A bilirubin above 25 mg/dl and a prothrombin time greater than 5 seconds above control are indicators of a poor prognosis. Long-term survival is improved by abstinence, but cirrhosis can still supervene, especially if severe inflammation and fibrosis were noted on liver biopsy.

The mainstays of treatment for alcoholic hepatitis, as for fatty liver, are abstinence and supportive care. A number of drugs have been evaluated in an effort to ameliorate the condition and to improve survival, including corticosteroids, D-penicillamine, propylthiouracil, and insulin plus glucagon. To date no agent has shown a consistently beneficial effect. Good nutrition is important; however these patients are often anorectic and may be encephalopathic. In patients with a tendency to encephalopathy, a vegetable protein diet (high in branched-chain versus aromatic amino acids) should be used. A multivitamin and folate may be given, but iron should be withheld unless iron deficiency is documented. It tends to accumulate in the liver and may potentiate liver damage. Vitamin K should be given parenterally as needed.

c. Cirrhosis. Cirrhosis is the end stage of alcoholic liver damage. Histologically, it tends to be micronodular. The signs and symptoms, complications, and treatment are similar to those of cirrhosis secondary to other etiologies. In one study, the 5-year survival was 63% in nondrinkers and 40.5% in continued drinkers. Jaundice, ascites, and hematemesis worsen the prognosis. If a patient lives beyond 2 years and continues to abstain, survival rates approach those for age-matched controls. Colchicine may be helpful in improving survival (1).

d. Hepatocellular Carcinoma. Hepatocellular carcinoma is discussed in II.G.2.9.

2. Drugs. A number of drugs have been noted to cause chronic liver damage in different histologic patterns.

a. Chronic Active Hepatitis. In general, the syndrome resembles autoimmune chronic active hepatitis clinically and histologically. Eosinophils may be present. It can lead to cirrhosis. The condition is more common in women and may manifest "autoimmune markers." α-Methyldopa causes chronic hepatitis in a small percentage of patients. The hepatitis improves on drug withdrawal, although scarring and cirrhosis remain. Isoniazid (INH) can cause chronic hepatitis if the drug is continued in a patient with acute hepatitis. Nitrofurantoin taken chronically (6 months to years) can cause chronic hepatitis, which resolves slowly on drug withdrawal. Oxyphenisatine, a laxative no longer available in the United States but still used in other parts of the world, causes chronic hepatitis, sometimes after years of usage. Usually drug withdrawal improves the condition, but on occasion it may progress nonetheless. Propylthiouracil and acetaminophen have been implicated in chronic hepatitis.

b. Other Histologic Lesions. Amiodarone and perhexilene maleate (an antianginal drug no longer available) cause phospholipidosis with an alcoholic hepatitis-like picture including Mallory bodies, which can progress to cirrhosis. Methotrexate, used for psoriasis as well as leukemia, can cause fibrosis. So can hypervitaminosis A in which there is hypertrophy of the Ito cells (perisinusoidal lipocytes), which store the Vitamin A. Chlorpromazine can cause a cholestatic lesion resembling primary biliary cirrhosis. 2'-Deoxy-5-fluorouridine infused into the hepatic artery as treatment for hepatic metastases can cause biliary sclerosis with jaundice, similar to sclerosing cholangitis.

3. Total Parenteral Nutrition (TPN). Mild elevations in aminotransferase and alkaline phosphatase activities are common in patients on TPN. Several specific syndromes are also seen. Excess calories given as carbohydrate can cause a tender fatty liver with small-droplet fat. The mechanism involves conversion of carbohydrate to triglyceride, which is then stored in the liver. Reduce the overall caloric intake and substitute lipid for some carbohydrate. Excess lipid can cause cholestasis. In infants, intrahepatic cholestasis, fibrosis, and cirrhosis can develop with prolonged TPN. Finally, TPN seems to predispose to formation of gallbladder sludge and gallstones, possibly secondary to bile stasis.

C. Metabolic Causes of Chronic Liver Disease

1. Nonalcoholic Fatty Liver. Fat can accumulate in the liver secondary to a variety of causes other than alcohol: obesity, diabetes mellitus, hypertriglyceridemia, corticosteroid therapy, jejunoileal bypass, protein malnutrition, parenteral hyperalimentation, drugs (valproic acid, intravenous tetracycline), Reye's syndrome, and fatty liver of pregnancy. The liver plays an important role in lipoprotein metabolism, taking up free fatty acids, synthesizing triglycerides, incorporating them into very low density lipoprotein (VLDL), and releasing VLDL into the bloodstream. Defects at a number of steps can lead to net hepatic fat accumulation. Histologically, the condition ranges from scattered droplets to extensive sheets of hepatocytes stuffed with lipid squeezing the cytoplasm into a thin rim. This can be reversed if the underlying cause is removed. Hepatocellular necrosis and inflammation around the terminal hepatic venules (central veins) is more dangerous and may lead to cirrhosis in a small percentage of cases. Necrosis may vary independent of fat. Mallory bodies may also be seen. Microvesicular fat, a distinct histologic picture, is seen in Reye's syndrome, fatty liver of pregnancy, and with intravenous tetracycline and valproic acid.

Clinically, the patient may be asymptomatic or complain of right upper quadrant discomfort. Hepatomegaly ranges from absent to marked. Liver tests may be normal or exhibit mildly elevated AST, alkaline phosphatase, and γ-glutamyltransferase (GGT) activities. Reye's syndrome and fatty liver of pregnancy are characterized by fulminant hepatic failure. A sonogram can confirm a suspicion of fatty liver. A liver biopsy may be done to investigate unexplained hepatomegaly. Treatment of a fatty liver in obesity or diabetes mellitus consists of weight reduction with emphasis on a low-carbohydrate diet.

2. Iron Overload. The general term "iron overload" includes idiopathic hemochromatosis, as well as the abnormal accumulation of iron secondary to other conditions. Normal iron homeostasis is maintained by a complex balance between iron losses, intestinal absorption, and iron stores (bone marrow, liver). Idiopathic hemochromatosis is an inborn error of metabolism inherited as an autosomal recessive. The frequency of heterozygotes (carriers) is 10–15% with homozygotes being 1 in 200–400. Approximately 20% of homozygotes develop clinical disease. Relatives of patients often have milder degrees of iron overload. Human lymphocyte antigens HLA-A3, -B14, and -B7 are increased in frequency. The precise defect is unclear, although patients seem to absorb inappropriately large amounts of iron relative to their (high) tissue stores. The disease is more common in males, presumably because females lose iron through pregnancy and menstruation. Patients present between 40 and 60 years of age, reflecting the many years required to accumulate sufficient tissue iron to affect organ function. Full-blown disease includes cirrhosis, diabetes, skin pigmentation ("bronze diabetes"), and heart failure. Joint involvement and hypogonadism are often present. In some patients, alcohol intake and dietary iron influence development of symptoms.

In the liver, hemosiderin granules (degraded ferritin) are deposited first in hepatocytes near portal areas and in bile duct epithelium. Kupffer cells are less involved. Mild or early cases may appear normal or exhibit portal tract fibrosis; advanced cases show cirrhosis. Hepatocellular carcinoma develops in 15–30% of patients and may supervene despite iron removal.

The diagnosis of idiopathic hemochromatosis may be suspected on clinical grounds. An unexplained elevation in AST, especially in a male, warrants a screen for the disease.

The plasma iron concentration is usually over 200 µg/dl (normal 80–180 µg/dl). The transferrin is fully saturated; however, technical difficulties in measurement may yield a saturation of only 60–70%. The plasma ferritin may be over 1000 ng/ml. Computed tomography (CT) scan can assess hepatic density and estimate the degree of iron overload. Liver biopsy can (a) estimate amount of iron; (b) measure actual amount of iron (requires special handling—consult a pathologist before biopsy); (c) assess pattern of iron deposition (parenchymal versus reticuloendothelial); and (d) assess degree of liver injury and fibrosis.

Relatives should be screened with plasma ferritin and transferrin saturation measurements. The importance of identifying individuals at risk prior to the onset of clinical disease cannot be overemphasized. HLA testing may be helpful.

Treatment involves removal of excess iron by venesection. With total body iron stores of 20–40 grams and 200 mg of iron present per pint of blood, weekly venesection therapy can take several years. Monitor plasma ferritin as a measure of remaining tissue stores. Once excess iron is removed, repeat phlebotomy every 2–3 months. Chelators like desferrioxamine require parenteral administration and remove only small amounts of iron. Reserve them for patients who cannot tolerate venesection.

Alcoholic cirrhosis is the most important of the secondary causes of iron overload. Liver biopsy shows less marked iron staining. Patients with hypoplastic anemia accumulate iron with repeated transfusions. Patients with thalassemia, refractory sideroblastic anemias, and pyridoxine-responsive anemias may accumulate iron with or without transfusions because of increased intestinal absorption stimulated by ineffective erythropoiesis. Iron overload may follow years of self-induced or iatrogenic (but inappropriate) oral iron therapy. Dietary exposure to excess in South African blacks ("Bantu siderosis") was caused by iron containers used to home-brew alcoholic beverages and by iron cooking pots.

3. Wilson's Disease. Wilson's disease (hepatolenticular degeneration) is an inborn error of metabolism resulting in depo-

sition of copper first in the liver, and then in the brain, corneas, and kidneys. As copper builds up in these organs over years, the signs and symptoms of disease appear. The condition is fatal if untreated. The exact defect is unknown but seems to be related to diminished biliary copper excretion. The incidence is approximately 1 in 33,000. The disease is inherited as an autosomal recessive, with a gene frequency (carrier rate) of approximately 1 in 100. The disease must always be considered in pediatric patients or young adults with otherwise unexplained liver disease. The presentations of Wilson's disease are protean. Liver manifestations range from acute hepatitis to chronic active hepatitis to cirrhosis. Signs and symptoms of liver disease vary according to the degree of pathology present. Consequently, these range from normal liver test results to mild elevations in aminotransferase activity, (with or without hepatosplenomegaly), through cirrhosis with portal hypertension and hepatic failure. On occasion, Wilson's disease may present as fulminant hepatic failure that can be fatal. Conversely, an initial attack may be self-limited, such that a patient presenting with cirrhosis may give a past history of "acute hepatitis" which in retrospect was a manifestation of Wilson's disease. Neurologically, a Parkinson-like tremor and rigidity may be seen, as well as drooling, a speech defect, and chorea. Behavioral changes are common. Other findings include hemolytic episodes (Coombs' test negative) or chronic hemolysis, calcified pigment gallstones, bone and joint symptoms, proteinuria, and decreased glomerular filtration rate (GFR). The characteristic eye finding is the Kayser-Fleischer ring, a deposit of copper in Descemet's membrane circling the iris. It is not, however, pathognomonic of Wilson's disease, having been described in primary biliary cirrhosis and familial intrahepatic cholestasis. Kayser-Fleischer rings are sometimes seen with the naked eye, but a slit-lamp exam is definitive. The ring may be absent in solely hepatic disease but is always present with neurologic disease. It may or may not be present in presymptomatic disease. Another, rarer eye feature is the sunflower cataract.

Several tests are used concomitantly in the diagnosis of

Wilson's disease. Serum copper concentration should be low and urinary copper excretion high, especially after a dose of chelating agent. The serum ceruloplasmin concentration should be low. Ceruloplasmin is a serum protein containing copper. It is the only oxidase circulating in the blood and is not the gene product of the defective gene in Wilson's disease. Look for Kayser-Fleischer rings on slit-lamp exam. On occasion, confusion can arise because ceruloplasmin can be low in heterozygotes and normal in homozygotes. Sometimes comparison of ceruloplasmin levels among parents (obligate heterozygotes), patient, and siblings can clarify the situation. In any event, all family members should be screened for the disease. In questionable cases, other tests may be useful, including staining for copper on routine liver biopsy, measurement of hepatic copper levels, and scans using radio-labeled copper. If the diagnosis is being considered, check with a pathologist concerning handling of the liver specimen prior to performing a biopsy.

Chelation is the mainstay of therapy for Wilson's disease. Penicillamine is most commonly used, but a multitude of side effects may preclude its use. Trientine (triethylene tetramine) may be substituted. Treatment must be continued for life. In rapidly progressive or unresponsive cases, liver transplantation should be considered.

4. α-1-Antitrypsin Deficiency. α-1-Antitrypsin is a protease inhibitor that protects cells from damage by trypsin and other proteolytic enzymes. Deficiency of α-1-antitrypsin is associated with liver and/or lung disease in some individuals. The mechanism is unclear, and it is not known why some are spared. There are at least 30 alleles at the protease inhibitor (Pi) locus. Genetically normal people have two M alleles (Pi MM). Homozygotes with the Z allele (Pi ZZ) account for approximately 1 in 2000 live births. Twenty percent present with neonatal cholestasis. Children with the Pi ZZ phenotype may develop cirrhosis early (by age 10) or later (by age 20); they may survive to adulthood with liver dysfunction, or may appear unaffected. In children, only homozygotes are noted to have liver disease. Some have lung disease as well. In adults, both cirrhosis and emphysema have been seen in homozygotes and heterozygotes.

The Pi MZ heterozygote has a 3% frequency (approximately 1 in 33 live births).

α-1-Antitrypsin deficiency may be suspected on serum protein electrophoresis (SPEP) by a decreased α-1-globulin band, since α-1-antitrypsin is the major component. Obtain a serum α-1-antitrypsin level. People with the Pi ZZ phenotype have only 10–15% of the normal level. Heterozygotes have an intermediate level. Protease inhibitor phenotyping can definitively establish the homozygous or heterozygous state. On liver biopsy, periodic acid-Schiff (PAS) positive, diastase-resistant inclusions are seen in periportal hepatocytes and sometimes in bile ducts. They may be present in homozygotes or heterozygotes, with or without liver disease and with or without emphysema. Similar inclusions can be seen in other disease states. There is no specific therapy for α-1-antitrypsin deficiency. Liver transplantation may be promising.

5. The Porphyrias. The term porphyria denotes a number of conditions representing enzyme defects (hereditary or acquired) in the biosynthesis of heme. Each defect causes accumulation of a different pattern of precursors in the pathway. They are classified into erythropoietic, hepatic, and erythrohepatic categories. Congenital erythropoietic porphyria does not affect the liver. There are four hepatic porphyrias: acute intermittent porphyria (AIP), hereditary coproporphyria (HCP), variegate porphyria (VP), and porphyria cutanea tarda (PCT). The first three (AIP, HCP, VP) are similar clinically, with acute attacks of abdominal pain, peripheral neuropathy, and psychiatric symptoms. Attacks may be precipitated by drugs (barbiturates, anticonvulsants, contraceptives), alcohol, fasting, and infection. Inheritance is autosomal dominant. Urinary porphobilinogen (PBG) and δ-aminolevulinic acid (δ-ALA) are elevated in acute attacks. The Watson-Schwartz test is a qualitative urinary PBG determination that requires a level three to five times normal to be positive. Between attacks, or in latent cases, diagnosis may be difficult, and sophisticated enzyme determinations may be necessary. In HCP, as the name implies, large amounts of coproporphyrin III are present in the feces and lesser amounts in urine. VP is characterized by

large amounts of protoporphyrin in the feces, with smaller amounts of coproporphyrin in feces and urine. HCP and VP may have cutaneous manifestations, as does porphyria cutanea tarda (see below). Liver tests results are normal or minimally abnormal. Treatment of an acute attack of AIP, HCP, or VP consists of intravenous glucose (20 g/hour) and/or intravenous hematin, as well as supportive care. Avoidance of precipitating factors is important.

The fourth hepatic porphyria, porphyria cutanea tarda (PCT), is the most common. It is characterized by chronic skin lesions: fragility and blistering with poor healing and scar formation, especially on light-exposed skin. Increased hair growth, especially on the face, is common. Liver disease is present. Patients do not manifest acute abdominal/neuropsychiatric attacks.

PCT may be hereditary (probably autosomal dominant) or acquired. Alcohol plays a role in some patients, and there is often iron deposition in the liver. Acquired PCT may be triggered by estrogen and polychlorinated hydrocarbons. There is an increased incidence of systemic lupus erythematosus (SLE), hemolytic anemia, and hepatocellular carcinoma. Urinary uroporphyrin is elevated, as is urinary coproporphyrin to a lesser degree. PBG and ALA are normal (which may explain the lack of neurological symptoms). Treatment consists of the elimination of alcohol and other possible precipitating factors, and phlebotomy. Sunscreens are not effective.

Protoporphyria (PP) is an erythrohepatic porphyria characterized by solar urticaria (burning and tingling on exposure to light) and solar eczema (cutaneous thickening on repeated exposure). Mechanical fragility and blistering are rare. It is inherited as an autosomal dominant trait. The liver may be involved even to the point of cirrhosis. There are no neuropsychiatric symptoms. The diagnosis is made by noting high levels of free erythrocyte protoporphyrin (FEP). ALA, PBG, and urinary porphyrins are normal. Treatment consists of oral β-carotene. Sunscreens are ineffective.

6. Other Inborn Errors of Metabolism. A variety of inborn errors of metabolism can affect the liver. Most are rare and are usually seen in children, many of whom die at an early

age. They usually represent defects in single enzymes. Some cause hepatitic deposition ("storage") of undegradable metabolites. There are disorders of tyrosine metabolism, carbohydrate metabolism, lipid metabolism, and the urea cycle. Disorders of carbohydrate metabolism include galactosemia; hereditary fructose intolerance; and the glycogen storage diseases, e.g., von Gierke's disease, Pompe's disease, and McArdle syndrome. Disorders of lipid metabolism include abetalipoproteinemia; the lipidoses; the sphingolipidoses (e.g., Gaucher's disease, Niemann-Pick disease, Tay-Sachs disease, Fabry's disease, and metachromatic leukodystrophy); and the mucopolysaccharidoses (e.g., Hurler's disease, Hunter's disease). In some cases, enzyme determinations or electron microscopy of liver tissue aids in diagnosis.

7. Benign Familial Recurrent Cholestasis. This syndrome presents as episodes of cholestasis with jaundice and pruritus without an obvious underlying cause. It may be present in several family members. The serum alkaline phosphatase and bile acids are elevated. Cholangiography demonstrates patent intrahepatic and extrahepatic bile ducts. Liver biopsy reveals bile plugs. Spontaneous remission occurs, but the condition is recurrent. Between attacks, liver tests and histology are normal. The disease does not progress to cirrhosis.

8. Liver Disease in Sickle Cell Anemia. Jaundice and liver disease may occur in sickle cell anemia via several mechanisms. Vascular occlusions in the liver secondary to sickle cells may cause hepatic infarcts. These may become infected, forming an abscess. The hemolytic anemia itself causes jaundice and a tendency to form gallstones. The gallstones may cause cholecystitis (difficult to distinguish from an abdominal crisis) and/or choledocholithiasis. These may be indications for surgery, but asymptomatic gallstones are not. Multiple transfusions introduce the risk of (chronic) hepatitis and liver damage secondary to iron overload.

D. Immunologic Causes of Chronic Liver Disease
   1. Primary Biliary Cirrhosis. Primary biliary cirrhosis (PBC) is a destructive disease of the small bile ducts of the liver. The etiology is unknown, although current theory favors an im-

munologic mechanism. It occurs mainly in women between the ages of 35 and 65, although 10% of the cases have been noted in males and in younger and older patients. The annual incidence is 5–10 per million, with a prevalence of one in 25,000.

The onset of disease is often insidious. An elevated alkaline phosphatase activity may be noted prior to onset of symptoms. Pruritus is the most common initial complaint. A small percentage of patients have evidence of advanced disease at the time of presentation. Xanthelasma and xanthomata may be present. Scratching may cause excoriations and a "butterfly" pattern of hyperpigmentation on the back.

The diagnosis is suggested by finding elevated alkaline phosphatase and γ-glutamyltransferase activities as well as the presence of anti-mitochondrial antibodies (AMA) in the appropriate clinical setting. Serum aminotransferase activities may be mildly elevated but proportionately less so than that of alkaline phosphatase. The bilirubin tends not to rise until the final stage of disease. Once it does, it is a sign of a poor prognosis. The serum immunoglobulin M (IgM) is elevated. Serum cholesterol may be elevate to >600 mg/dl in a few cases. Visualize the biliary tree via endoscopic retrograde cholangiopancreatography (ERCP) to rule out bile duct disease, including sclerosing cholangitis. Perform a liver biopsy. Four stages are noted histologically: (*a*) active bile duct destruction with infiltration by lymphocytes and plasma cells, usually with granulomas; (*b*) ductular proliferation, sometimes with lymphoid aggregates where bile ducts had been, and with variable piecemeal necrosis merging into (*c*) scarring and (*d*) cirrhosis. Bile plugs, copper, and Mallory bodies may be noted in periportal hepatocytes.

The disease tends to progress to cirrhosis over approximately 5–10 years. A few patients may live as long as 20 years after diagnosis. In addition to pruritus and fatigue, osteoporosis (and osteomalacia) may occur. Several diseases with presumptive immunologic mechanisms may be seen concurrently, including Sjögren's syndrome, scleroderma, rheumatoid arthritis, autoimmune thyroiditis, SLE, and the CREST syndrome (calcinosis, Raynaud's phenomenon, esophageal involvement, sclerodactyly, and telangiectasia).

The complications of cirrhosis are treated in the usual manner. Plasmapheresis can decrease serum cholesterol and shrink xanthomata. While no treatment is universally accepted, there are studies in support of colchicine (0.6 mg b.i.d.) and of methotrexate. The former in particular should be considered because it is so well tolerated. At present, liver transplantation is recommended when the disease reaches its final stages.

2. Autoimmune Chronic Active Hepatitis. First described by Waldenstrom in 1950, autoimmune chronic active hepatitis (AICAH) was known early on as "lupoid hepatitis." We now know it is unrelated to systemic lupus erythematosus, although it also occurs mainly in young women. Symptoms may be absent or vary from mild to severe fatigue, with all the complications of cirrhosis. The diagnosis is suggested by the presence of smooth muscle antibody (SMA) in the context of chronic hepatitis. The serum γ-globulin is greatly elevated and may be so high as to cause a hyperviscosity syndrome. Occasionally, non-A, non-B hepatitis or other conditions may manifest a low titer of smooth muscle antibody, but the globulin is not elevated and this is probably a nonspecific effect. Although not part of the diagnosis, lupus erythematosus (LE) cells are present in 10–15%. Mitochondrial antibody is absent. Aminotransferase activities range from near normal to approximately 700 units. There may be wide fluctuations without obvious cause. In severe cases, or at end stage, jaundice supervenes. On liver biopsy, the usual histologic features of chronic active hepatitis are present (see above). Parenchymal collapse is more prominent than in viral hepatitis. Active inflammation ranges from mild to severe, with or without cirrhosis. Biopsy results may not correlate with symptoms or lab values. Treatment is usually reserved for patients in whom more than one parameter (symptoms, laboratory values, histology) is severely abnormal, but experienced clinical judgment is required. Treatment consists of prednisone, usually 10–15 mg/day. Some use doses starting at approximately 40 mg/day, tapering slowly to 10–15 mg/day This does increase side effects. Some centers use prednisolone in equivalent doses. Azathioprine in doses of 50 mg/day may be added in hopes of decreasing the corticosteroid requirement. Recent British

experience indicates that azathioprine has benefits of its own, contrary to earlier studies. Planned treatment continues for at least 6 months (and sometimes up to several years) with the aim of decreasing ongoing hepatic necrosis and slowing progression to cirrhosis. It is not clear that the latter is achievable with current therapy. The decision to treat should be considered carefully, since: (a) it is prolonged; (b) it can cause major side effects; and (c) tapering the patient off corticosteroids may result in a worsening of symptoms and laboratory values, committing the patient to additional unplanned years of treatment. Patients with the hyperviscosity syndrome respond to plasmapheresis. At end stage, transplantation is indicated.

E. Vascular Causes of Chronic Liver Disease

    1. Chronic Passive Congestion. Congestive heart failure (CHF) can cause liver damage secondary to lack of oxygen at the cellular level. This process may be acute, chronic, or chronic with acute exacerbation. Cardiac etiologies include coronary artery disease, mitral stenosis, tricuspid regurgitation, and constrictive pericarditis. The patient may be asymptomatic or complain of right upper quadrant pain (more likely in an acute or acute on chronic process). The liver may be normal in size or enlarged to the umbilicus. Ascites, when present, may seem out of proportion to the degree of CHF. Although classically a transudate is expected, some patients manifest an exudate. Jaundice is usually mild, but bilirubin levels up to 26 mg/dl have been noted. Aminotransferase activities are mildly elevated in chronic passive congestion. They can reach up to 1000 units/L in acute conditions associated with hypotension and subsequent ischemic damage to the liver ("shock liver"). Aminotransferase activity can fall rapidly toward normal with treatment of the heart failure. This is equally true for the high levels associated with hypotension. On liver biopsy, zone 3 (around the central vein or terminal hepatic venule) is the most sensitive to hypoxia, since its usual blood supply is oxygen-poor relative to the other zones. Sinusoidal dilatation is common. Cardiac cirrhosis can result from long-standing right-sided heart failure. The chronically hypoxic central areas undergo necrosis and fibrosis. Gross examination demonstrates a

"nutmeg" liver with alternating red areas of congestion and pale areas of fibrosis.

2. Budd-Chiari Syndrome. Budd-Chiari syndrome results from occlusion of the hepatic veins and/or inferior vena cava. Etiologies include oral contraceptives, polycythemia vera, tumor invasion of the inferior vena cava (hepatocellular carcinoma, hypernephroma), fibrous web (probably congenital), and paroxysmal nocturnal hemoglobinuria. The syndrome presents with right upper quadrant pain (secondary to a large, tender liver) and ascites. Jaundice, if present, is mild. If the vena cava is involved, collaterals appear on the abdomen and back. Portal hypertension develops, with all its complications. Right-sided heart failure is absent. Diagnosis may be difficult. Standard liver test results are nonspecifically abnormal. The ascitic fluid protein may be high. Liver-spleen scan sometimes shows increased uptake centrally, possibly due to hypertrophy of the caudate lobe. This lobe drains directly into the vena cava and may not be involved.

Hepatic vein catheterization may yield useful information but is technically difficult in these patients. Vena cavography should be done first. Liver biopsy shows centrilobular congestion and sinusoidal dilatation. Webs can be dilated surgically or with a balloon. Treatment of other conditions is unsatisfactory. Peritoneoatrial shunting may be palliative. Transplantation offers some hope.

3. Venoocclusive Disease. Venoocclusive disease involving the smallest hepatic veins and venules causes a syndrome clinically similar to the Budd-Chiari syndrome. It can result from ingestion of pyrrolizidine alkaloids ("bush tea"), other herbal teas, especially comfrey, radiation to the liver, and chemotherapeutic agents.

F. Congenital Causes of Chronic Liver Disease

1. Caroli's Disease. This syndrome consists of congenital focal cystic dilatation of the intrahepatic bile ducts, often in association with congenital hepatic fibrosis. The main consequence is recurrent attacks of bacterial cholangitis, which may present as unexplained fever. The diagnosis is suspected on sonography or computed tomography. Although cholangiography demonstrates the lesion well, it may pre-

cipitate cholangitis. Alkaline phosphatase and GGT activities may be moderately elevated. Cholangitis is treated with antibiotics. In some patients, recurrent cholangitis is suppressed (if not prevented) by prophylactic antibiotics. Biliary-intestinal anastomosis risks increasing attacks of cholangitis. Segmental disease may be treated by partial hepatectomy. Liver transplantation may be considered for poorly controlled recurrent cholangitis in a patient with diffuse disease.

2. Congenital Hepatic Fibrosis. Congenital hepatic fibrosis is a hereditary condition (autosomal recessive), which causes portal hypertension. Histologically, the hallmark is marked enlargement of portal spaces with fibrosis and bile ductular proliferation. The ducts may form microcysts, which may or may not communicate with the biliary tree. Regenerative nodules are not present. Associated conditions include Caroli's disease (see above) and dilatation of renal collecting tubules, sometimes with renal cysts.

Clinically, the disease often presents with variceal bleeding, usually between the ages of 5 and 20 years. Liver function is normal. Liver biopsy demonstrates the lesion noted above: however, there may be sampling error, since not all portal spaces are involved. Variceal hemorrhage should be treated with sclerotherapy.

G. Neoplastic Causes of Chronic Liver Disease
1. Benign.
   a. Adenomas. Hepatic adenomas are benign tumors seen most commonly in women taking oral contraceptives or men using anabolic steroids for muscle building for many years. They present as a right upper quadrant mass with or without pain, or occasionally as hemoperitoneum after rupture. Histologically the lesion consists of plates of hepatocytes more than one or two cells thick. Since Kupffer cells are absent, adenomas do not take up technetium on liver scan. Although the lesions may regress on discontinuation of the medication, surgery may be considered for large lesions.
   b. Focal Nodular Hyperplasia. Histologically a hamartoma, focal nodular hyperplasia has a characteristic appearance grossly, with a central stellate scar. The lesion is more

common in women. Oral contraceptives cause the lesion to enlarge and occasionally bleed. Most cases are found incidentally at surgery. Occasionally a mass is palpable, but usually they are asymptomatic and rarely bleed.

c. Cysts. Hepatic cysts can be solitary or multiple, small or quite large. They are sometimes discovered as an incidental finding on sonography or computed tomography. They are generally asymptomatic, although very large cysts can cause hepatomegaly and abdominal pain because of bleeding into the cyst. Rarely, a large cyst may rupture. Liver cysts may be associated with renal cysts (polycystic disease). Liver tests are normal. Treatment is generally not necessary. Occasionally, resection may be considered for very large symptomatic cysts. This can be quite difficult technically and should be reserved for life-threatening complications. Echinococcal cysts are considered above.

d. Hemangiomas. Hemangiomas are the most common benign lesion of the liver. They may be single or multiple, large or small. Like liver cysts, they may be discovered incidentally during sonography or computed tomography. When large, they may present with hepatomegaly. A dynamic liver scan or magnetic resonance imaging (MRI) may be helpful in diagnosis. Angiography confirms the diagnosis but is usually not necessary. Liver biopsy may lead to hemorrhage. Complications are rare, but include spontaneous hemorrhage and diffuse intravascular coagulation (DIC). Surgery is rarely indicated.

2. Malignant.

a. Hepatocellular Carcinoma. Hepatocellular carcinoma (HCC) is one of the most common malignant tumors worldwide. In the United States, HCC accounts for 1–2% of all malignancies. Approximately 75% of patients with HCC have cirrhosis of varying etiologies. Worldwide, hepatitis B is the most common associated factor. Hepatitis B viral DNA can integrate into the genome of liver cells, even in patients without (measurable) hepatitis B surface antigen. In addition to posthepatic cirrhosis (B or non-A, non-B), etiologies include alcohol, hemochromatosis, α-1-antitrypsin deficiency, and other diseases. Patients with these conditions or with chronic hepatitis should be monitored periodically with α-fetoprotein levels (see below) and sonograms. Patients with autoimmune chronic hepatitis or primary biliary cirrhosis rarely develop HCC.

HCC is more common in males than in females. Clinically, the disease may be silent, may present with painful hepatomegaly, or may cause sudden deterioration in a stable cirrhotic. A friction rub or bruit may be noted over the liver. The new onset of ascites may herald HCC and should be investigated. In a patient with cirrhosis, a space-occupying lesion on sonography or scanning is highly suspect, although sometimes these represent regenerative nodules. Routine liver test results may not differ from those of the underlying condition, or may exhibit more marked increases of alkaline phosphatase and GGT activities. Paraneoplastic manifestations (e.g., hypoglycemia, polycythemia) are prominent in occasional patients. α-Fetoprotein (AFP) is a useful marker for HCC. Levels up to 200–400 ng/ml may be seen in acute or chronic hepatitis with regeneration after hepatocellular injury. Levels higher than this, up to tens of thousands, are seen in HCC. Histologically, multiple tumor nodules are often seen. This has been cited as proof that HCC is multicentric; however intrahepatic metastasis is an alternate explanation. Fibrolamellar carcinoma is a variant of HCC found in young adults with underlying normal livers.

The diagnosis of HCC can be made clinically when a space-occupying mass and high AFP are noted in a cirrhotic patient. Poor clotting function may preclude obtaining a specimen of tissue. Percutaneous liver biopsy can yield a false negative result. It rarely causes bleeding, even if the lesion is very vascular. Needle track metastases are also rare. Sonography- or computed tomography-directed biopsy may be useful, although here, too, the lesion may be missed or the aspirate may not be diagnostic. Laparoscopy may be considered.

For the small percentage of patients in whom the tumor is small, hepatic resection may be attempted, although underlying cirrhosis may compromise the outcome. The majority of patients, however, die within 6 months of diagnosis. Chemotherapy, including infusion into the hepatic artery, has thus far not been very helpful. Patients with fibrolamellar HCC should undergo resection or liver transplantation.

b. Cholangiocarcinoma. Cholangiocarcinoma, carcinoma of bile duct origin, is less common than hepatocellular carcinoma. It may present at the hilum of the liver (as obstructive jaundice) or peripherally, with abdominal pain and nonspecific symptoms. Some patients show an association with ulcerative colitis, sclerosing cholangitis, or choledochal cysts. Although an attempt should be made to determine resectability, it is usually not possible. Treatment is largely palliative via insertion of drainage tubes or surgical decompression.

c. Angiosarcoma. This is a rare, rapidly progressive disease associated with several carcinogenic agents including vinyl chloride and thorium dioxide (thorotrast). The latter is a radioactive imaging agent no longer used, the effects of which are still being seen in patients who received it in the past. Epithelioid hemangioendothelioma is a related but less malignant variety, which can be treated by transplantation.

d. Metastatic Tumor. The liver is a common site for metastatic tumor deposits, especially from primary tumors in the lung, GI tract, pancreas, and breast; and from lymphoma and melanomas. Signs and symptoms referrable to the liver may be absent, or may include abdominal pain, hepatomegaly, jaundice, and ascites. At times cancer may present as metastatic disease before a primary tumor has been identified. No pattern of liver test abnormalities is specific for metastatic disease. Test results may be normal but are usually elevated (alkaline phosphatase more commonly, but aminotransferases as well). Jaundice results from massive hepatic replacement by tumor, and less commonly from duct obstruction except in Hodgkin's disease. Carcinoembryonic antigen (CEA) may be present in cancers of the GI tract, breast, and lung. The diagnosis is suggested on radiologic imaging (liver scan, ultrasound, or CT) and confirmed by biopsy (percutaneous, directed by ultrasound or CT, or laparoscopic). Treatment with chemotherapeutic agents is largely palliative. On occasion, a solitary metastasis is surgically resectable.

H. Other Causes of Chronic Liver Disease

1. Granulomas. Hepatic granulomas are caused by numerous etiologies, including infections (tuberculosis, atypical mycobacteria, histoplasmosis, schistosomiasis), sarcoidosis, hypersensitivity reactions to drugs and other agents, collagen vascular diseases, lymphoma, and various primary liver diseases. They may be an incidental finding of little diagnostic significance. Sometimes, they are discovered during evaluation of a systemic disease or a fever of unknown origin. Even so, it may be very difficult to discover the etiology (not found in 25%), and further diagnostic work-up depends on the clinical setting. Certain histologic features suggest particular etiologies, although usually granulomas of different origins look very similar. Caseating granulomas suggest TB. If this disease is suspected, submit a specimen of liver for culture and staining. (In general, examination of the bone marrow should be performed before a liver biopsy is done for TB). Of the noncaseating granulomas, sarcoidosis is characteristically periportal. Eggs may be noted in schistosomiasis. Symptoms are usually those of the underlying conditions, or may be absent. Half the patients have hepatomegaly. Liver test results may be normal or may demonstrate elevations of alkaline phosphatase and aminotransferase activities. Occasionally, liver test results may be quite abnormal, e.g., in some patients with sarcoidosis. Therapy consists of treatment of the underlying disease. Often no particular therapy is necessary. In those cases where symptoms, e.g., fever, persist and no specific etiology is discerned, a trial of antituberculous therapy is warranted, followed by a trial of corticosteroids.

2. Primary Sclerosing Cholangitis. This syndrome of inflammation and fibrosis of bile ducts of unknown etiology affects the intrahepatic and/or extrahepatic biliary tree. In the latter case it must be distinguished from cholangiocarcinoma, choledocholithiasis, biliary stricture (spontaneous or postsurgical), and other bile duct abnormalities. It is associated with

inflammatory bowel disease, usually ulcerative colitis, but also Crohn's disease in about two thirds of patients. The condition is more common in males and usually presents in the 25- to 45-year age range. Jaundice and pruritus may be intermittent initially but eventually become chronic. Other symptoms include pain and fever, the latter signaling cholangitis. Laboratory abnormalities include increases in alkaline phosphatase and GGT activities and possibly elevated bilirubin levels. The diagnosis is established by radiological visualization of the biliary tree in a patient without a history of bile duct surgery or stones. Endoscopic retrograde cholangiopancreatography (ERCP) is most useful, showing tortuous bile ducts with stenotic areas interspersed with beaded dilatations. Liver biopsy may show cholangitis, whorls of fibrous tissue surrounding and obliterating bile ducts (classic but difficult to demonstrate), and/or cirrhosis. Once the disease is diagnosed, look for inflammatory bowel disease if not previously suspected. The condition is progressive, causing secondary biliary cirrhosis with portal hypertension and liver failure. There is no accepted medical treatment. Methotrexate and cyclosporine are being tested. Cholestyramine may be used for pruritus and antibiotics for acute cholangitis. Surgical drainage of the biliary tree has been advocated in the past. However, prior biliary surgery (as well as sclerosing cholangitis itself) may technically complicate liver transplantation, the modality that is the major hope for these patients.

3. Secondary Biliary Cirrhosis. This condition results from mechanical obstruction of the biliary tree by a number of disorders: stricture (spontaneous or postsurgical), choledocholithiasis, chronic pancreatitis, extrinsic compression, sclerosing cholangitis, congenital biliary atresia, and cystic fibrosis. Patients with pancreatic or bile duct cancer generally do not live long enough to develop biliary cirrhosis. The condition takes from 3 months to 1 year to develop, but is seen in only a small proportion of patients with predisposing conditions. The precise role of infection in the bile is unclear. Jaundice, pruritus, and episodes of cholangitis are seen. Increases in alkaline phosphatase, GGT activities, and bilirubin levels are more pronounced than increases in

aminotransferase activities, although the latter may be moderately raised in acute cholangitis. Treatment consists of early decompression of the biliary tract, since cirrhosis will not be reversed.

4. Amyloidosis. The liver is commonly involved in amyloidosis, causing hepatomegaly but rarely liver failure or portal hypertension. Alkaline phosphatase activity may be elevated but does not correlate well with extent of infiltration with amyloid. Histologically, the amyloid material appears as homogenous pink deposits in the space of Disse. Primary amyloidosis often shows involvement of the walls of hepatic arterioles. The material demonstrates the characteristic green birefringence on Congo red stain. Although liver biopsy may be safely performed in amyloidosis to establish the diagnosis, more accessible organs should be biopsied first, since fractures of the liver have occurred.

5. Cryptogenic Cirrhosis. *Cryptogenic cirrhosis* is the term used to designate cirrhosis of indeterminate etiology. Although sometimes used interchangeably with *posthepatitic cirrhosis*, the latter term should be reserved for cases presumed secondary to viral hepatitis (B or non-A, non-B).

III. Complications of Cirrhosis

A. Portal Hypertension

The portal vein drains blood from the abdominal portion of the GI tract, spleen, pancreas, and gallbladder into the liver. Normal pressure is 5–10 mm Hg or 10–15 cm saline. Portal hypertension is defined as a wedged hepatic venous pressure (WHVP) > 4 mm Hg above pressure in the inferior vena cava, or an intraoperative portal pressure >30 cm saline. Ohm's law states that $V = IR$, i.e., the pressure in a rigid system equals flow × resistance. The law is not strictly applicable to the liver, since the portal circulation is not a rigid system. Nonetheless, the concept of a relationship between portal pressure, blood flow, and vascular resistance is still a useful one. Traditionally, the role of vascular resistance has been emphasized. Portal hypertension has been classified into presinusoidal (portal vein thrombosis, schistosomiasis), sinusoidal (cirrhosis), and postsinusoidal (Budd-Chiari syndrome, venoocclusive disease) "blocks." Conditions in which portal hypertension may be secondary to increased inflow include hematologic diseases with large spleens and splanchnic arteriovenous fistulae. The importance of blood flow on portal pressure has been underscored by the use of β-adrenergic blocking agents, which may decrease portal pressure by decreasing splanchnic blood flow.

To a large extent, the well-recognized complications of cirrhosis (esophageal varices, ascites, hepatic encephalopathy, splenomegaly with hypersplenism) are consequences of portal-systemic shunting due to portal hypertension.

B. Esophageal Varices and Other Collaterals
In portal hypertension, collaterals form where veins draining the high-pressure portal system anastomose with veins draining the lower-pressure caval system. Esophageal (and gastric) varices form by anastomoses between the coronary vein (portal drainage) and the azygos vein (superior vena cava drainage), possibly with a contribution from the perisplenic veins (portal) to the short gastric veins (caval). Hemorrhoidal anastomoses may occur between the middle and superior hemorrhoidal veins, which drain blood from the upper rectum into the portal system, and the inferior hemorrhoidal veins, which drain blood from the lower rectum into the inferior vena cava. Collaterals can form on the anterior abdominal wall between the umbilical vein remnant (portal) and the epigastric veins (caval). A "caput medusae" is formed when these vessels appear to radiate from the umbilicus. Indeed, blood does flow away from the umbilicus, i.e., upward above and downward below the umbilicus. Distinguish this from inferior vena cava obstruction, in which blood flow is upward below the umbilicus.

The presence of esophageal varices should be suspected in any patient with known liver disease or a clinical picture compatible with cirrhosis. It may be noted radiographically but is made with certainty endoscopically. Cirrhotic patients may bleed from lesions other than esophageal varices, including duodenal ulcers and gastritis. Since therapy for these conditions differs radically from therapy for bleeding varices, establishing the diagnosis of bleeding esophageal varices is crucial. The treatment of bleeding esophageal varices is discussed in chapter 3.

C. Ascites

1. Pathogenesis. Multiple factors are responsible for the formation of ascites in portal hypertension. They interact in a complex process, which has not been fully elucidated. There is increased production of hepatic lymph which cannot be accommodated by the lymphatics. The serum albumin level is usually considered important as well, i.e., the lower the albumin, the less the degree of portal hypertension necessary to produce ascites. Avid sodium retention is noted. Whether this is primary or secondary is unclear. If primary, increased blood volume, noted experimentally, causes "overflow" of ascites. In the traditional hypothesis, sodium retention is secondary to a low "effective" plasma volume, a putative volume smaller than the total blood volume, which the volume receptors sense to trigger aldosterone release. Aldosterone levels are high, but aldosterone is only part of the explanation. The role of the kidney and related hormones (including atrial natriuretic peptide) in the formation and maintenance of ascites is complicated and incompletely understood.

2. Clinical Considerations. Clinically, shifting dullness, a fluid wave, and bulging flanks may be noted. To detect small amounts of ascites, position the patient on hands and knees and percuss the "puddle sign" from below. Ultrasound is also useful to detect small amounts of fluid.

   The new onset of ascites necessitates a paracentesis for diagnosis. In cirrhosis the fluid is usually a transudate, although exudates may be seen with spontaneous bacterial peritonitis, hepatocellular carcinoma, and occasionally for reasons which are unexplained.

   See Table 9.2 for the differential analysis of ascitic fluid.

3. Treatment. The initial objective should be prevention. Ascites is far easier to prevent than to treat. Cirrhotics without ascites often develop it in the hospital as a result of overly vigorous intravenous hydration.

   In treating ascites, sodium intake must be restricted beyond the body's capacity to excrete sodium. The usual sodium restriction for cardiac disease is not sufficient. Restrict sodium intake to 200–500 mg/day. With severe ascites, especially with hyponatremia, restrict fluid to 750–1000 ml/

Table 9.2.
Differential Analysis of Ascitic Fluid[a]

Type of Ascites	Appearance	Protein (g/dL)		Leukocytes[b]			Cytology	Peritoneal Biopsy	Culture	pH	Amylase	Other
		Mean	Range	PMN[c]	MN	Total[d]						
Cirrhotic	Clear	1.8	0.6–6.0	75	225	300 ±400	0	NS	0	7.45	Normal	Occasionally turbid; rarely bloody
Cardiac	Clear	2.2	1.5–5.5	50	200	250 ±200	0	NS	0	7.40	Normal	Liver biopsy diagnostic
Neoplastic	Clear/bloody	2.2	0.6–6.0	340	360	700 ±300	+ (30%)	+ (50%)	0	7.35	Normal	Occasionally chylous
Bacterial peritonitis	Cloudy	1.0	0.6–2.2	2200	300	2500 ±2500	0	NS	+	7.25	Normal	Culture positive
Pancreatic	Clear/bloody	3.2	1.0–5.0	900	1000	1900 ±800	0	NS	0	7.38	Elevated (80%)	Occasionally chylous
Tuberculosis	Clear	3.4	1.5–7.0	125	875	1000 ±600	0	+ (65%)	+ (65%)	7.30	Normal	Occasionally chylous
Nephrotic	Clear	0.9	0.3–1.8	45	175	220 ±200	0	0	0	7.38	Normal	
Postdialysis	Clear	1.3	1.0–3.0	50	200	250 ±200	0	0	0	7.40	Normal	

[a]From Conn H, Atterbury CE: Cirrhosis. In Schiff L, Schiff ER (eds): *Diseases of the Liver.* Philadelphia, JB Lippincott, 1987, p 770. Reprinted with permission of Dr. H. Conn.
[b]Mean per mm³
[c]PMN, polymorphonuclear leukocytes; MN, mononuclear cells; NS, nonspecific; 0, negative; +, positive.
[d]Mean ± SD.

day. Bed rest improves renal clearance. Spironolactone is usually the first diuretic used. Start with a dose of 50 mg b.i.d. Weigh the patient daily. Measure abdominal girth. The goal is weight loss of approximately 0.5 kg/day. More may be mobilized if peripheral edema is present. Urinary sodium and potassium may also be used to monitor response. In untreated cirrhotics, urinary sodium (Na^+) excretion is low and potassium (K^+) excretion is higher. Look for a reversal of this urinary Na^+/K^+ relationship, i.e., urinary Na^+ excretion should rise, while the K^+ excretion falls. If there is no response, double the dose in 3–5 days, up to a total of 400 mg. Tender gynecomastia develops in many male patients early in therapy, making continued use unacceptable. Response to thiazides is poor in cirrhosis. Often furosemide (Lasix) must be added (or used alone) to obtain diuresis. Begin with a dose of 40–80 mg. Up to 240 mg of furosemide may be used. Intermittent therapy (twice per week) is more effective than daily therapy.

Large-volume paracentesis (removal of 4–6 liters) has recently come back into vogue. Albumin may or may not be infused intravenously. The procedure may be used for respiratory embarrassment. Note that the presence of massive ascites per se is not an indication for therapeutic paracentesis. Care should be taken not to precipitate hypotension and/or the hepatorenal syndrome, as is also true for diuretics.

Water immersion is an experimental technique that results in natriuresis. Although results are interesting, it is not widely available at present. Peritoneovenous shunts (Le Veen, Denver shunts) extract fluid from the peritoneal cavity and reinfuse it into the venous circulation. Although complications include infection, blockage of the tube, and DIC, shunts can be quite useful in about two-thirds of patients.

D. Hepatic Encephalopathy
  1. Clinical Presentation. Hepatic encephalopathy (portal-systemic encephalopathy) is a condition of altered mental status related to hepatic dysfunction. It varies from subtle changes detectable only via psychometric testing to frank coma. Encephalopathy is graded 1–4.

Grade 1 (mild): tremor, impaired handwriting;

Grade 2 (moderate): asterixis, impaired computation, lethargy;

Grade 3 (severe): confusion, somnolence;

Grade 4 (coma): responsiveness to painful stimuli, present initially, is lost as coma deepens.

2. Pathogenesis. The pathogenesis of hepatic encephalopathy is not well understood, although there are several hypotheses. Multiple factors are probably important.

   a. Ammonia Hypothesis. It is unlikely that ammonia, per se, is causative, but it is a useful place to begin discussion. Ammonia produced in the gut by ingestion of protein and bacterial metabolism is carried to the liver via the portal vein. In cirrhosis, portal-systemic shunting of blood diverts ammonia from the liver, where it would be metabolized to urea, to the systemic circulation, where toxic levels are reached. Several facts must be kept in mind:

      i. Blood ammonia levels do not correlate with degree of encephalopathy, although arterial levels may correlate better than venous levels.

      ii. Most patients with cirrhosis have chronically high ammonia levels with or without encephalopathy.

      iii. The ammonia level may rise 1–2 days before clinical symptoms appear and drop before clinical improvement occurs.

   b. Amino Acid Hypothesis. Blood levels of aromatic amino acids (AAA) (tyrosine, tryptophan, phenylalanine) are elevated in hepatic encephalopathy, while levels of branched-chain amino acids (BCAA) (leucine, isoleucine, valine) are lowered. Aromatic amino acids may be precursors of false neurotransmitters in the central nervous system (CNS), while BCAAs block entry of AAAs into the CNS.

   c. γ-Aminobutyric Acid (GABA) Hypothesis. GABA is an inhibitory neurotransmitter in the central nervous system. Elevated levels are found in hepatic encephalopathy. However, it does not appear to be the only mediator of encephalopathy noted in cirrhosis.

   d. Fatty Acid Hypothesis. Short chain fatty acids (butyric, valeric, octanoic) have been implicated.

    e. Benzodiazepine Receptor Hypothesis. This hypothesis is favored at present. A receptor that binds benzodiazepines has recently been recognized in proximity to the GABA receptor. There are early reports of short-term reversal of hepatic encephalopathy by an experimental agent (flumazenil) working at this site. While this work is very exciting, further investigation is necessarv to determine its full significance.

3. Precipitating Factors. Many factors can precipitate encephalopathy, either alone or in concert. These include: a protein load, whether dietary or secondary to blood in the GI tract; constipation; azotemia, including that produced by diuretics; hypokalemia; sedatives; sepsis; and alkalosis.

4. Treatment. Treatment of hepatic encephalopathy consists of the following:

    a. Correct the precipitating factors. If patient is constipated, give a tap water enema. Discontinue sedatives and diuretics.

    b. Remove blood and/or protein from the GI tract with cathartics and/or enemas. Lactulose is a nonabsorbable disaccharide, which works in several ways. It causes diarrhea, is metabolized by colonic bacteria to acidify luminal contents and convert NH_3 to unabsorbed NH_4^+, and alters gut flora. The initial dose is 30 ml orally, t.i.d. Larger doses can cause severe diarrhea and electrolyte imbalance. Titrate the dose to produce 2–3 soft stools/day. If necessary, give lactulose as an enema (60 ml lactulose in 500 cc water).

    c. Neomycin may be added in unresponsive cases, but care should be used in renal insufficiency. The usual dose is 1 gram orally b.i.d., but a higher dose (6 g/day for two days) may be used initially to achieve a rapid response.

    d. Diet should consist of vegetable protein only (to favor branched-chain amino acids versus aromatic amino acids).

    e. Good supportive care is essential, e.g., vitamins, prevention or treatment of infection, and *judicious* use of intravenous fluids, since most patients already have ascites and edema. Do not use hypotonic solutions, since these worsen dilutional hyponatremia.

E. Spontaneous Bacterial Peritonitis

This is a condition usually occurring in patients with chronic liver disease and ascites. Note that the signs and symptoms of peritonitis, e.g., abdominal pain, fever, and leukocytosis, may be absent. While culture of bacteria from the fluid is diagnostic, therapy must often be instituted prior to the results of ascitic fluid culture becoming available. The most common organisms are *Escherichia coli*, *Klebsiella*, *Streptococcus pneumoniae*, and *S. faecalis*. In many patients, the culture is negative but a clinical response to antibiotics is noted. Inoculation of ascitic fluid into culture medium at the bedside (including anaerobic medium) may increase the yield. An important factor in the decision whether to treat is the ascitic fluid cell count. More than 500 polymorphonuclear neutrophils (PMNs) per mm^3 or more than 1000 leukocytes/mm^3 are indications to treat even in the absence of symptoms. Broad spectrum antibiotics are used initially and modified once culture results are available. Avoid aminoglycosides.

F. Hepatorenal Syndrome

This condition of renal failure in the setting of cirrhosis and ascites carries a high mortality. It is characterized by progressive azotemia and oliguria often triggered by diuresis or paracentesis. Other cases include GI bleeding and sepsis. The pathogenesis is unknown, although altered renal hemodynamics and possibly prostaglandins may play a role. The kidneys themselves are normal and have been used for kidney transplantation. Treatment is seldom successful. Occasionally volume expansion with albumin or peritoneovenous shunting may be helpful, but no more than 1 liter of normal saline and 1–2 units of albumin should be given.

G. Hypersplenism

Splenomegaly (an enlarged congested spleen) may be seen in patients with portal hypertension. It can cause significant pancytopenia secondary to sequestering of formed blood elements (hypersplenism). Splenectomy is rarely indicated for hypersplenism secondary to liver disease and may jeopardize subsequent transplantation. If liver disease is absent, other causes of splenomegaly must be ruled out.

H. Other Complications

Cirrhosis can cause a coagulopathy on several bases. The liver is involved in synthesis of most of the coagulation factors. Even factor VIII, which is generally felt to be nonhepatic, may have a small procoagulant portion that is synthesized by the liver. Circulating fibrinogen may be decreased. Fibrin split products are sometimes seen signalling low-grade DIC. The prothrombin time is often elevated. This may be due to hepatocellular dysfunction; however, in cholestasis, lack of bile in the GI tract causes deficiencies of the fat-soluble vitamins A, D, E, and K. Administer vitamin K (10 mg subcutaneously every day for three days). An improvement in prothrombin time implies that obstruction to flow of bile, rather than hepatocellular dysfunction, was the problem. Thrombocytopenia secondary to hypersplenism is often present. Vitamin D deficiency contributes to metabolic bone disease, e.g., in PBC.

REFERENCES

1. Kershenobich D et al.: Colchicine in the treatment of cirrhosis of the liver. *New Engl J Med* 318:1709–1713, 1988.
2. Hoofnagle JH, et al.: Randomized, controlled trial of recombinant human α-interferon in patients with chronic hepatitis B. *Gastroenterology* 95:1318–1325, 1988.

SUGGESTED READINGS

Schiff L, Schiff ER (eds): *Diseases of the Liver*. Philadelphia, JB Lippincott, 1987.
Wright R, Millward-Sadler GH, Alberti KGMM, Karran S (eds): *Liver and Biliary Disease*. London, Ballière Tindall, WB Saunders, 1985.

Chapter 10

Diarrhea
Jacob S. Walfish, M.D.

I. **Approach to the Patient**

  A. Introduction

    Diarrhea is defined as the presence of more than 250 cc of water in the stool per day. When a patient presents with a chief complaint of diarrhea, he or she is aware that there has been a change in bowel habits, but the description of the problem may be otherwise quite vague. Before trying to diagnose a cause for "diarrhea," the physician should have a clear idea of the patient's present "abnormal" and past "normal" habits.

    1. The frequency, consistency, amount, and timing of the patient's movements, and the overall duration of the complaint should be ascertained. Problems of urgency and incontinence ("accidents") need to be asked about explicitly.

    2. For poor historians, obtain a stool chart documenting the frequency and content of stool.

  B. Associated Symptoms

    1. Symptoms related to the gastrointestinal (GI) tract, including abdominal pain, nausea, vomiting, GI bleeding, and perianal disease, can help localize the site of disease. Enteritis is often accompanied by bloating, periumbilical pain, nausea, and vomiting. Colitis may produce localized left-sided pain and rectal bleeding.

    2. Systemic symptoms such as fever, weight loss, arthritis,

and flushing, as well as known systemic disease such as diabetes, cardiovascular disease, scleroderma, and immune deficiency, together with related drug treatment must all be explored.

C. Other Historical Data
Travel, sexual, drug, and family history may all provide important clues.

II. Acute Diarrhea

A. Diarrhea of Infectious Origin
Sudden onset of loose or watery stools in a previously healthy person is usually of infectious etiology, especially if there is associated fever and abdominal cramping. Supportive history includes a viral prodrome, recent travel history, synchronous onset of symptoms in friends or family, or recent ingestion of contaminated food or water (food poisoning).

B. Organisms
A wide variety or organisms, including bacteria, viruses, and protozoa (see Chapter 12) may cause acute diarrhea. However, a specific diagnosis, which sometimes requires extensive stool laboratory studies, is often unnecessary when the illness is mild and self-limited.

C. Laboratory Features
1. Work-up for a specific pathogen should be carried out under the following conditions:
   a. Bloody stools (if bleeding from a hemorrhoid or fissure has been excluded).
   b. Immunocompromised host.
   c. Clinical dehydration or toxicity.
   d. Progressive or persistent symptoms for more than 5 days.
2. If microbiologic studies are indicated, send fresh specimens for specific studies. Avoid contamination by barium, Kaopectate, or Pepto Bismol. When specific organisms are suspected, communicate directly with the laboratory. Thus, if blood or pus suggest inflammatory diarrhea, alert the lab to search for invasive organisms such as *Campylobacter, Salmonella, Shigella, Yersinia, Pleisiomonas,* and *Entamoeba histolytica.* A recent travel history would suggest agents endemic to the area visited.

3. Prior antibiotic use should prompt an assay for *Clostridum difficile*, and a history of "food poisoning" would lead to suspicion of *Vibrio, Clostridia, Staphylococcus, bacillus cereus,* and their toxins. Noninflammatory acute diarrhea is often due to viral agents, including adenovirus, enterovirus, and the Norwalk agent. However, the latter are usually diagnosed by exclusion after pathogens such as *Giardia* and *Aeromonas* are ruled out.

4. Homosexual males must be screened for the organisms known to cause the "gay bowel syndrome," and AIDS patients must be investigated for a broad range of common and opportunistic infections.

D. Drug-Induced Diarrhea

Drug-induced diarrhea is easily diagnosed but frequently overlooked. Possible offenders include antacids, laxatives, antibiotics, nonsteroidal anti-inflammatory agents, diuretics, quinidine, and colchicine. Review the manufacturer's list of side effects for each medication taken by the patients. However, when a temporal association suggests drug-induced diarrhea, consider a drug withdrawal trial even if diarrhea has not been a reported side effect. In patients with malignancy, suspect acute iatrogenic diarrhea from chemotherapy or radiotherapy.

E. Paradoxical Diarrhea

Paradoxical diarrhea may result from acute partial small bowel obstruction, usually in association with crampy pain, or from stool impaction and overflow incontinence in the elderly patient. Plain x-rays of the abdomen and rectal exam may be sufficient for diagnosis in such cases.

III. Chronic Diarrhea

A. Introduction

Chronic diarrhea is often a more difficult diagnostic problem. Since many of the agents that cause acute diarrhea may also cause chronic diarrhea, they should be reliably excluded before embarking on an extensive diagnostic work-up.

B. Functional Diarrhea

Although so-called functional diarrhea or diarrhea due to "irritable bowel syndrome" is a diagnosis of exclusion, a presumptive diagnosis can often be made on the basis of the history, physical examination, and simple blood screening. Chronic, nonprogressive symptoms in the absence of nocturnal symptoms, weight loss, fever, anemia, or blood in the stool, should raise the possibility of functional diarrhea. If the patient is young, relates symptoms to stress, and has palpable tubular sigmoid colon, a therapeutic trial for irritable bowel syndrome is warranted, especially if there are intercurrent periods of constipation. Since lactase deficiency may produce a similar picture, a trial of lactose-restriction would also be indicated in this setting. However, in the older patient, a colonic neoplasm must always be excluded early on by barium enema or colonoscopy before making a diagnosis of irritable bowel syndrome, which rarely has its initial onset in older age.

C. Basic Pathophysiologic Mechanisms
When organic disease is suspected, systematic evaluation should be guided by the suspected pathophysiologic mechanism. The basic mechanisms can be classified as follows:

1. Osmotic Diarrhea. Caused by poorly absorbable, osmotically active solutes that lead to retention of water in the lumen.
2. Hypersecretory Diarrhea. Due to increased electrolyte secretion by the small or large bowel.
3. Malabsorptive Diarrhea. Due to decreased absorption of fluid, electrolytes, or nutrients.
4. Inflammatory Diarrhea. Due to structural damage with exudation of blood and pus in the stool.
5. Diarrhea due to abnormal motility of the small or large bowel.

D. Multiple Pathophysiologic Mechanisms
In specific diseases, multiple pathophysiologic mechanisms may be operative. In many forms of infectious diarrhea, for example, hypersecretion, mucosal inflammation, and altered motility may all coexist. Inflammatory bowel disease may cause malabsorptive as well as inflammatory diarrhea. Nevertheless, certain generalizations based on this classification are useful:

1. Diarrhea that is purely due to hypersecretion, hyperosmotic substances, or altered motility should not cause blood or pus in the stool; conversely, the presence of blood or pus implies bowel inflammation or ulceration.

2. Caveats.
    a. When there is blood in the stool, always exclude a hemorrhoid or fissure that may complicate any diarrheal state.
    b. Mild colonic mucosal hyperemia seen on sigmoidoscopy and microscopic inflammatory changes on mucosal biopsy are often nonspecific and may be found with diarrhea of any cause.
3. Hyperosmolar and malabsorptive diarrhea will improve in the fasting state; hypersecretory diarrhea will not. Response to fasting will be variable in diarrhea due to inflammation.
4. Significant diarrhea in the absence of weight loss is unlikely to be due to malabsorption.
E. Specific Causes for Chronic Diarrhea
The following are specific causes for chronic diarrhea classified by pathophysiologic mechanism:
    1. Osmotic Diarrhea.
        a. Laxative abuse using magnesium sulfate or phosphate compounds, or saline cathartics (always suspect in chronic, difficult-to-diagnose cases, particularly in women prone to eating disorders such as anorexia nervosa or bulimia).
        b. Disaccharidase deficiency including lactase, and isomaltose-sucrase deficiency (sorbitol, found in chewing gum, is poorly digestible and may cause diarrhea).
    2. Hypersecretory Diarrhea.
        a. Laxative abuse with castor oil, phenolphthalein, cascara, etc.
        b. Hormonally medicated pancreatic cholera, WDHA (watery diarrhea, hypochlorhydria, and acidosis) syndrome), Zollinger-Ellison syndrome, medullary carcinoma of the thyroid, carcinoid syndrome, ganglioneuroma.
        c. Secretory villous adenoma.
        d. Bile-salt induced.
    3. Malabsorption (see Chapter 11).
        a. Intestinal disease—tropical and nontropical sprue, Whipple's disease, abetalipoproteinema, intestinal lymphangiectasia, inflammatory bowel disease.
        b. Maldigestion due to pancreatic disease, biliary obstruction, bacterial overgrowth, bile salt deficiency.
        c. Anatomic causes—surgical bypass, postgastrectomy, short bowel, fistula.

      d. Other causes—infectious (giardiasis, cryptosporidiosis); lymphoma.

4. Inflammatory Diarrhea.
      a. Infections.
      b. Inflammatory bowel disease.
      c. Neoplasms—carcinoma, lymphoma.
      d. Radiation- or chemotherapy-induced enteritis.
      e. Ischemia.

5. Altered Motility.
      a. Irritable bowel syndrome.
      b. Systemic disease, including hyperthyroidism, diabetes mellitus, scleroderma (with bacterial overgrowth).
      c. Postsurgical, including postgastrectomy or postvagotomy, blind loop, chronic partial bowel obstruction due to adhesions.
      d. Drug-induced (see comments on acute diarrhea).
      e. Stool impaction with fecal incontinence.

F. Diagnostic Tests

Although the list of diagnostic tests available for evaluation of diarrhea is quite long (Table 10.1), a detailed history guided by the pathophysiologic principles outlined above should minimize the number of tests required to make a diagnosis. In general, simple tests on stool and blood should precede more complex radiologic or invasive procedures. Sigmoidoscopy should be considered an extension of the physical examination and should be performed promptly when the possibility of rectosigmoid disease exists.

G. Collagenous and Microscopic Colitis

1. These newly recognized entities should be considered when the usual evaluation for chronic diarrhea is unrevealing. They are much more common in women than in men.

2. Watery diarrhea may be persistent or intermittent and may be variably associated with weight loss or crampy abdominal pain. Stool shows no blood or inflammatory cells.

3. Barium enema and colonoscopy are either entirely normal or show nonspecific changes. However, mucosal biopsies show excessive acute and chronic inflammatory cells, occasional cryptitis, and sometimes thickening of the subepithelial collagen band.

Table 10.1.
Diagnostic Investigations for Evaluation of Diarrhea

Investigation	Findings
Stools	
Gross examination (may confirm but sometimes contradicts a patient's description)	Solid, loose, watery, bloody
Microscopic examination	Occult blood, pus, undigested fat, organisms
Culture (always be specific and communicate directly with lab, if possible)	Pathogenic organisms
Toxin assay	*C. difficile* toxin
Laxative assay	Specific laxatives; phenolphthalein
	Laxatives give pink color with alkalinization
24-hour volume and weight (regular diet and fasting)	If volume >500 cc, organic disease is likely, irritable bowel syndrome is unlikely
	If volume decreases significantly with fasting, suspect osmotic or malabsorptive diarrhea
24–72 hour collection for fat (on 100-g fat diet)	>6 g fat per day suggests fat malabsorption
Stool electrolytes and osmolarity (applicable only to liquid stools)	Osmotic gap suggests ingestion of osmotic laxatives
Blood	
Hemoglobin	Microcytic anemia-blood loss, macrocytic anemia-malabsorption
White blood cell count	May be elevated with infection or IBD*
Electrolytes	Hypokalemia and acidosis occur in secretory diarrhea
Serum proteins	May be low in malabsorption, neoplasm, and protein-losing enteropathy
β-carotene, calcium, folate, vitamin B_{12}	Low in malabsorption

Table 10.1. (continued)
Diagnostic Investigations for Evaluation of Diarrhea

Blood	
Amylase	Sometimes elevated with pancreatitis or pancreatic neoplasm
Thyroxine (T$_4$)	Hyperthyroidism
Gastrin	Z-E syndrome
VIP, calcitonin levels	Pancreatic cholera, medullary carcinoma of the thyroid
Serology	Amoebiasis, *Yersinia*, HIV infection
Serum immunoglobulins	Immunoglobulin deficiency syndromes

Urine	
Screen for laxatives	Phenolphthalein gives pink color with alkalinization
5-HIAA	Carcinoid

Radiology	
Plain film of abdomen	Dilated bowel suggestive of chronic obstruction or pseudo-obstruction
	Ahaustral colon suggestive of chronic ulcerative colitis
	Pancreatic calcification with chronic pancreatitis
Upper GI small bowel series (always obtain complete study with spot film of the terminal ileum)	"Malabsorption pattern," dilated, edematous bowel, rapid transit with fistula or short bowel
	Neoplasms—lymphoma, carcinoid, ileitis, or jejunitis (A normal study does not always exclude small bowel disease)
Barium enema	Colitis, neoplasm (a normal study does not always exclude colitis)

Other Studies	
Abdominal sonogram, CT scan	Pancreatic tumor (glandular or islet cell tumor)
Fiberoptic colonoscopy	Gross and microscopic colitis

Table 10.1. (continued)
Diagnostic Investigations for Evaluation of Diarrhea

Biopsy for histology and culture	Specific infection—CMV, herpes, TB, and atypical mycobacteria
Small bowel biopsy (endoscopic or blind)	Sprue, Whipple's disease, lymphoma, giardiasis
D-Xylose absorption test	If normal, valuable in excluding malabsorption due to mucosal disease
Lactose tolerance hydrogen breath test	Useful in cases of questionable lactase deficiency
$^{14}CO^2$ breath test with ^{14}C-glycocholate	May detect bile salt deconjugation
Secretin test	Abnormal in pancreatic insufficiency

[a]IBD, inflammatory bowel disease; Z-E, Zollinger-Ellison; VIP, vasointestinal peptide; CMV, cytomegalovirus; TB, tuberculosis; 5-HIAA, 5-hydroxyindole acetic acid.

4. There is no proven therapy; however, spontaneous resolution may occur. Sulfasalazine, steroids, loperamide, and psyllium mucilloid may be of benefit in some cases.

SUGGESTED READING

Dobbins JW, Binder HS: Pathophysiology of diarrhea, alteration in fluid and electrolyte transport. *Clin Gastroenterol* 10:605–625, 1986.

Chapter 11

Malabsorption Syndromes
Charles D. Gerson, M.D.

I. Introduction

A. Definition

Malabsorption is a broad descriptive term that encompasses many different diseases. In general, the syndromes of malabsorption are manifested by increased fecal excretion of ingested nutrients, often including fat. For this reason, the term *malabsorption* is often used synonymously with *steatorrhea*, or increased stool fat. This usage, however, is incorrect, since not all malabsorption syndromes produce steatorrhea and since steatorrhea is not always attributable to malabsorption. Technically, *malabsorption* refers to abnormal mucosal transport of one or more specific substances. This abnormality is different from *maldigestion*, which refers to abnormal intraluminal events. In common clinical parlance, however, derangements of mucosal transport and of intraluminal digestion are both described as "malabsorption syndromes."

B. The Absorption Process

There are several steps in the process of absorption.

1. The intraluminal phase includes solubilization of ingested material. This can be abnormal due to several factors, including:

   a. Inadequate mixing of enzymes and food.

   b. Pancreatic insufficiency.

   c. Inadequate bile concentration.

2. The mucosal phase relies on an adequate absorptive surface, and mucosal diseases, including enzyme deficiencies of the brush border, can cause a failure of mucosal absorption.
3. The removal of nutrients from the gut is the last phase of absorption and can be abnormal due to obstruction of vascular or lymphatic flow. Lymphatic drainage is necessary for fat absorption, while carbohydrates and proteins are carried away in the venous system. Diseases that block lymphatic flow, such as tuberculosis, lymphoma, and lymphangiectasia, can all lead to failure of nutrient removal.

C. Fat Malabsorption

Fat malabsorption will be discussed as an example.

Maldigestion of fats can be secondary to either impaired lipolysis or impaired micelle formation. Impaired lipolysis can be secondary to poor mixing (postgastrectomy patient), altered lipase (Zollinger-Ellison syndrome inactivating lipase secondary to a low pH), and inadequate amounts of lipase (pancreatic insufficiency). Impaired micelle formation can occur secondary to a lowered bile-salt pool (liver disease, biliary obstruction, ileal disease), or altered bile salts (bacterial overgrowth leading to deconjugation).

Fat malabsorption can be due to multiple causes such as decreased contact time with the absorptive surface (fistula, jejunoileal bypass intestinal resection), abnormal mucosal surface (sprue, ischemia, radiation), decreased chylomicron formation abetalipoproteinemia), and decreased transport (Whipple's disease, lymphoma, lymphangiectasia).

II. Approach to the Patient

A. History
1. The hallmarks of a malabsorption syndrome are weight loss, diarrhea, and evidence of a nutrient deficiency. These are not always obvious in the early stages, and there is certainly a clinical spectrum, which may begin with only one of the above manifestations.
   a. Weight loss may be gradual rather than acute in presentation. It is important to realize that patients may not appear to have lost weight, especially if they were obese at the onset of their disease. Patients with malabsorption

      also may note that they lose weight in spite of a good appetite with normal or high caloric intake.

  b. Most patients with malabsorption do not have prominent complaints of abdominal pain.

  2. It is important to differentiate small bowel-induced diarrhea from colon-induced diarrhea. While the rule is not infallible, a history of frequent watery movements usually means colon-induced diarrhea, whereas less frequent, semi-formed, bulky stools suggest small bowel origin. Bloody diarrhea is unusual in malabsorption, and it points to a colonic source. Floating, greasy stool is classically described in steatorrhea, but it is seldom observed.

B. Physical Examination

  1. Examination revealing evidence of weight loss, as well as specific nutrient deficiencies, can help in the evaluation of the patient with malabsorption. The presence of ecchymoses points to a vitamin K deficiency, hyperkeratosis to vitamin A deficiency, and peripheral edema to hypoalbuminemia; tremors or tetany can point to calcium or magnesium deficiencies. Examination of the tongue can show the pallor and glossitis of folic acid or vitamin B_{12} malabsorption.

  2. In addition to the manifestations above, patients with malabsorption may have mild to moderate abdominal distention. This is caused by small intestinal dilatation, not by ascites, and is often in contrast to the effects of weight loss on the rest of the body. In most patients with malabsorption, there will be no abdominal tenderness, just as there will not be a complaint of abdominal pain.

C. Laboratory Features

  1. Blood Tests.

    a. Hemoglobin can be low. This finding can be a marker for either lack of iron, or folate and vitamin B_{12} absorption. The mean corpuscular volume (MCV) may be helpful, unless there is a combined deficiency; in this case, red blood cell distribution width index (RDW) may be high. An elevated MCV may be the first sign of malabsorption, usually caused by folic acid deficiency.

    b. Cholesterol. In most patients with malabsorption, especially if steatorrhea is present, serum cholesterol will be quite low (often below 150 mg/100 ml).

c. Carotene. This precursor of vitamin A is useful as a screening measure, and should be below 30 mg/100 ml. Any patient with profound malnutrition from any cause may also have a very low serum cholesterol and carotene.

d. In patients with advanced malabsorption, depressed levels of calcium, magnesium, and albumin, and an elevated prothrombin time may also be observed. The abnormal prothrombin time should be correctable by parenterally administered vitamin K. Serum levels of iron, B_{12}, and folate can be obtained routinely.

2. Tests of Absorption.

a. Stool analysis can be either qualitative or quantitative. Examination of the stool, using a Sudan stain on a random stool sample for the presence of fat droplets and undigested muscle fibers, can suggest that malabsorption is occurring. The classic 72-hour fecal/fat collection, while difficult and unpleasant, is still the "gold standard" for the diagnosis of steatorrhea. It is important that the patient be able to take in about 80–100 grams of fat per day for the test to be valid.

Steatorrhea is defined as fat excretion greater than 7 g/24 hours on a diet of 80–100 g/day.

b. An x-ray of the small intestine can reveal a number of abnormalities associated with malabsorption. Changes specific for sprue, Crohn's disease, and jejunal diverticulosis, as well as infiltrative disease of the small intestine, can be seen with this technique.

c. The D-xylose test evaluates mucosal integrity by testing carbohydrate absorption. D-Xylose is a pentose only partly metabolized by human beings. Twenty-five grams are given by mouth. Sixty percent of the ingested dose is absorbed in the duodenum and proximal jejunum in normal people, and about 20% of the absorbed dose is excreted in the urine within 5 hours. A D-xylose level in a 5-hour urine collection greater than 5 grams is normal. A level of less than 2.5 grams, in the presence of normal renal function and in the absence of ascites, is indicative of diffuse mucosal disease in the duodenum and proximal jejunum. If renal function is impaired, then a 2-hour blood sample can be obtained instead of urine collection, with a serum level of less than 30 mg/dl being abnormal. The test is also abnormal in cases of bacterial overgrowth, since bacteria metabolize the xylose. Other causes of falsely abnormal results are incomplete ingestion of the xylose, vomiting, and delayed gastric emptying.

d. The Schilling test is useful not only in diagnosing vitamin B_{12} malabsorption but also in determining its cause. Normally, ingested B_{12} binds preferentially to R proteins in the acid milieu of the stomach. Intrinsic factor is released by the antrum; and within the duodenum, pancreatic enzymes digest away the R proteins, leaving B_{12} free to bind to intrinsic factor. The B_{12}-intrinsic factor complex is absorbed within the ileum. Thus, one needs a working stomach, pancreas, and ileum for normal B_{12} absorption to take place. During the Schilling test, B_{12} is initially given parenterally to load all the body's binding sites, so that all intestinally absorbed B_{12} will be excreted in the urine. B_{12} bound to a radioactive marker (cobalt-57) is given by mouth, and urine is collected. B_{12} absorption is abnormal if B_{12} is not found in the urine. To isolate a specific cause of malabsorption, there are several manipulations that can be undertaken. B_{12} bound to intrinsic factor and labeled with cobalt is given by mouth to determine if malabsorption is secondary to lack of intrinsic factor. The test can be repeated with pancreatic enzymes, as well, to determine if malabsorption is secondary to pancreatic insufficiency. The test can be repeated with antibiotics to treat bacterial overgrowth to determine if this was the cause of malabsorption.

e. Small intestinal biopsy can be obtained in several ways. Currently, two methods are considered the methods of choice: suction biopsy with small bowel biopsy tubes passed orally under fluoroscopy, and endoscopically obtained biopsy. It is important that the biopsy be obtained from the region of the duodenal-jejunal junction so as to avoid normal mucosal flattening due to Brunner gland hyperplasia found within the duodenum. Small bowel biopsy can be diagnostic in patients with celiac sprue, tropical sprue, intestinal lymphoma, Whipple's disease, and lymphangiectasia.

f. There are several available breath tests to document bacterial overgrowth or lactose intolerance. In the bile acid breath tests, the patient is given a radioactively labeled bile salt. If increased amounts of radioactive carbon dioxide are found in the breath, then there is either small bowel bacterial overgrowth, or less absorptive ileal surface with bacterial deconjugation of bile salts in the colon. A breath hydrogen test uses no isotopes and can also document bacterial overgrowth. Normally, only small amounts of hydrogen are found in exhaled air. With bacterial overgrowth, ingested glucose reaches the small intestine, where bacterial degradation leads to hydrogen formation. Similarly, patients with lactose intolerance have increased breath hydrogen after a dose of lactose, since the lactose is metabolized by bacteria in the colon. This is a highly sensitive measure of lactase deficiency.

g. In a lactose tolerance test, a patient is given 50 grams of lactose by mouth, and blood glucose levels are monitored. Lactase deficiency is likely when glucose levels do not rise more than 20 mg/100 ml over a 2-hour period.

III. Specific Disorders of Malabsorption

A. Postgastrectomy

A common cause of mild malabsorption is a Billroth II operation. This can lead to an afferent loop syndrome, with stasis and bacterial overgrowth of both aerobic coliforms and anaerobes. In addition, rapid entry of nutrients into the jejunum results in inefficient mixing with digestive juices, often leading to mild steatorrhea. Digestive enzymes from the pancreas are not released appropriately because secretin and cholecystokinin (CCK), which are more concentrated in the lamina propria of the duodenum, are not released when food goes directly into the jejunum. Finally, iron and calcium absorption may be impaired, since the main site of their absorption, the duodenum, is bypassed. Medical treatment includes intermittent antibiotics and supplementation with calcium and iron. Treatment is usually empiric, and consists of periodic treatment depending on the symptoms. A typical example is a 7-day course per month of an antibiotic; agents such as tetracycline, metronidazole, and trimethoprim-sulfamethoxazole may be rotated monthly. More severe cases of afferent loop syndrome may require revision of the anastomosis.

B. Bacterial Overgrowth

Bacterial overgrowth causes fat malabsorption due to bile-salt deconjugation and resultant poor micellar formation. Any cause of stasis of intestinal contents can lead to bacterial overgrowth. Possible mechanisms include:

1. Decreased motility due to diabetes, scleroderma, and pseudoobstruction syndrome.
2. Blind loop due to surgery, fistula.
3. Partial small bowel obstruction due to Crohn's disease.
4. Small bowel diverticula.

C. Celiac Sprue

This is the prototype of malabsorption syndrome, though it should be remembered that it is primarily a disorder of the jejunum, not the ileum. It appears to be caused by an immunologic reaction to gluten, the protein in wheat, rye, barley, and oats. This reaction is mediated via T lymphocytes in the lamina propria and may be genetically influenced, since there is increased prevalence of certain histocompatibility antigens such as HLA-B8 and HLA-DW3. There is an association between sprue and a skin condition, dermatitis herpetiformis. Patients with the latter also have a high prevalence of HLA-B8. Some patients will have a history of wheat intolerance during infancy and childhood, but the majority will have the onset beginning in the 3d or 4th decade. Presentation will be either the typical malabsorption syndrome with features of steatorrhea, or a more subtle form of the disorder, with deficiency of just one important nutrient, such as iron. Sprue is suggested by a low D-xylose test, and small bowel dilatation on x-ray. Definitive diagnosis, however, requires the finding of subtotal villous atrophy on small bowel biopsy. Since the treatment is lifetime and the differential diagnosis extensive, biopsy is essential in every case. After the diagnosis is made by small bowel biopsy, primary treatment is adherence to a gluten-free diet. While clinical response may occur within a week or two, it often takes months before absorption parameters and biopsy return toward normal. Since patients with sprue usually have a secondary lactase deficiency, avoidance of lactose-containing foods may be helpful. If a patient does not respond to dietary treatment, there can be several possible reasons, including erroneous diagnosis, inadvertent gluten ingestion, refractory sprue, hypogammaglobulinemia, sprue with giardiasis, and small intestinal lymphoma. Refractory sprue may be only partially refractory, and these patients can respond to the addition of steroids. If the condition is totally nonresponsive, as in collagenous sprue, the use of extreme measures such as home parenteral hyperalimentation may be necessary.

D. Tropical Sprue

This occurs mainly in two areas of the world, the Indian subcontinent and the Caribbean, although it may be found elsewhere in the developing world. People who come from those areas may develop tropical sprue after migration to a temperate climate. There are several features that distinguish tropical sprue from celiac sprue. Tropical sprue involves both the jejunum and ileum, while celiac sprue involves only the proximal small bowel. The main feature of tropical sprue is megaloblastic anemia, rather than steatorrhea as in celiac sprue. Most patients with tropical sprue respond to a 2- to 6-month course of folic acid and tetracycline. Tetracycline is used because a number of gram-negative organisms have been found in the small intestine of affected patients. There is no one specific bacterium responsible for this disease.

E. Whipple's Disease

This is a rare cause of malabsorption, with three main symptoms: diarrhea, fever, and arthritis. It primarily affects males. The cause is bacterial, and a small, gram-positive organism can be identified microscopically in the lamina propria. Breakdown of these organisms results in the typical finding of periodic acid-Schiff (PAS)-positive macrophages, the hallmark of Whipple's disease. Treatment is with long-term antibiotics such as penicillin and trimethoprim-sulfamethoxazole.

F. Intestinal Lymphangiectasia

This is a rare disease manifested by dilated lacteals in the lamina propria of the small intestinal villi, and associated with impaired absorption of fat. It is the classic example of a protein-losing enteropathy, as proteinaceous material actually leaks from the lacteals into the intestinal lumen. Peripheral edema is the major manifestation, and treatment consists of a low-fat diet plus supplementation of the diet with medium chain triglycerides, which can be absorbed directly into the bloodstream.

G. Radiation Enteritis

This complication may occur in patients who have received large doses of radiation therapy, usually exceeding 5000 rads. It is common after treatment of gynecologic malignancy, especially in patients who have had abdominal surgery prior to radiation, so that a fixed segment of small bowel was repeatedly exposed. It is usually a late complication occurring years after the radiation. Symptoms can be due to a stricture with partial small bowel obstruction, fistula formation, or occasionally a significant protein leak. Treatment obviously depends on the segment and length affected, and may consist of nutrient supplements. Occasionally, resection or bypass of a diseased segment may be required.

H. Small Bowel Resection

Resection of the small intestine may cause significant malabsorption, depending on which segment, and how much is removed. Most of the problems occur in patients who have had ileal resection, especially of the terminal ileum. The degree of malabsorption will depend on whether or not more than 90 cm has been removed. This is the critical length of resection for significant bile salt depletion with resultant steatorrhea. With less than 90 cm removed, excess bile salts may enter the colon and produce choleretic diarrhea, but the liver will compensate with sufficiently increased synthesis of bile salts to be adequate for fat absorption. In this case, treatment with the bile salt binding resin, cholestyramine, will be effective.

SUGGESTED READINGS

Trier JS: Diagnostic value of peroral biopsy of the small intestine. *New Engl J Med* 285:1470, 1971.

Olson WA: A pathophysiologic approach to diagnosis of malabsorption. *Am J Med* 67:1007, 1979.

Falchuk ZM: Gluten-sensitive enteropathy. *Am J Med* 67:1085, 1979.

Chapter 12

Infectious Diarrhea (Including AIDS)

Lawrence B. Cohen, M.D.
Peter H. Rubin, M.D.

NON-AIDS-RELATED INFECTIOUS DIARRHEA

I. **Overview: Infectious Diarrhea**

A. Causes
May be caused by viruses, bacteria, and protozoans (Table 12.1).

B. Prognosis
In developed countries, most cases resolve without specific therapy, although worldwide, infectious diarrhea is a major cause of morbidity and mortality.

C. Predisposing Factors
More likely in patients who have:
1. Achlorhydria.
2. Impaired intestinal motility (e.g., scleroderma, postradiation, diabetes, postsurgery, blind loops, and small intestinal diverticulosis).
3. Immunocompromise.
4. Malnutrition.
5. Poor hygiene.
6. History of travel or antibiotic use.

Table 12.1.
Prominent Causes of Infectious Diarrhea and Their Differentiating Features

Organism	Source	Incubation Period	Clinical Features	Positive Culture
S. aureus	Creamy pastries, potato salad meat, milk products	2–6 hours	Vomiting; explosive, nonbloody diarrhea	No
Toxigenic E. coli	Water	1–3 days	"Travelers diarrhea"—watery, explosive onset; nausea; chills; cramps	No
V. cholerae	Water, crabs, shrimp	6–48 hours	Abrupt, explosive "rice water" stool; severe fluid and electrolyte depletion; no abdominal pain or fever	Yes*
C. botulinum	Improperly canned fruits and vegetables, and smoked fish	1–8 days	Vomiting; cranial neuropathy (diplopia, dysarthria, dysphagia	Yes*
C. perfringens	Beef, poultry	None	Cramps; sudden, explosive, nonbloody diarrhea	Yes*
V. parahemolyticus	Undercooked or raw seafood, shellfish	12–48 hours	Headaches; explosive, watery diarrhea with cramps and vomiting	Yes
B. cereus	Chinese rice and vegetables	1–16 hours	Vomiting and abdominal pain *or* diarrhea	Yes
Shigella	Contaminated food, water or infected humans	24–48 hours	Early watery and then bloody diarrhea; tenesmus	Yes

Table 12.1. (continued)
Prominent Causes of Infectious Diarrhea and Their Differentiating Features

Organism	Source	Incubation Period	Clinical Features	Positive Culture
Salmonella	Poultry, meat eggs, dairy products, and infected humans	6–48 hours	Watery or bloody diarrhea with or without systemic symptoms	Yes
Campylobacter	Unpasteurized milk, infected animals, contaminated meat, humans	3–5 days	Prodrome of headaches, malaise, myalgias, fever; bloody diarrhea	Yes[a]
C. difficile	Antibiotics	4 days–6 weeks	Profuse watery diarrhea; fever; abdominal pain; leukocytosis	Yes (toxin)
Giardia	Water	12–15 days	Nausea; epigastric distress; flatulence; nonbloody diarrhea	No[b]
Amoeba	Anal-oral	Variable	Variable, from no symptoms to nonbloody to severe, bloody diarrhea.	No[b]

[a]Not identified by standard stool culture procedures. When suspected, laboratory must be notified.
[b]May be diagnosed by microscopic analysis.

D. Differential Diagnosis
   1. Idiopathic inflammatory bowel disease (ulcerative colitis and Crohn's disease).
   2. Other toxins (e.g., chemical, heavy metal, marine, mushroom).
   3. Hormonal excess (e.g., gastrinoma, pancreatic tumors, hyperthyroidism, carcinoid).
   4. Malabsorptive or maldigestive states (e.g., celiac sprue, tropical sprue, chronic pancreatitis).
   5. Drug-induced diarrheas (e.g., quinidine, colchicine).

II. Pathogenesis

A. Enterotoxin Production
   1. Usually food-borne and either ingested as preformed toxin or toxin produced in vivo.
   2. Toxins act as secretagogues.
   3. The mucosal surface of the gastrointestinal (GI) tract is not physically violated.
   4. Diarrhea is typically watery and voluminous.
   5. There is usually no septicemia and little, if any, fever.
   6. Microscopic analysis of stool reveals no leukoctyes or organisms.
   7. Examples: Cholera, toxigenic *Escherichia coli*, *Clostridium perfringens*, *Staphylococcus aureus*.

B. Mucosal Invasion
   1. Microorganisms invade the GI lining, interfering with normal absorptive processes.
   2. These organisms may also elaborate enterotoxins and increase local synthesis of prostaglandins.
   3. Typically, the resultant diarrhea is bloody, mucoid, and sometimes of low volume, with associated tenesmus.
   4. There may be associated fever, arthritis, rash, and septicemia.
   5. Leukocytes are present on microscopic analysis of stool.
   6. Examples: *Shigella*, *Salmonella*.

C. Miscellaneous
   1. Many of the infectious diarrheal agents appear to be both enterotoxic and invasive. Examples: *Campylobacter*, some species of *E. Coli*.

2. *Clostridium difficile* produces a necrotizing cytotoxin, resulting in colitis.
3. Rotavirus, Norwalk virus, and strains of adenovirus invade the small bowel mucosa, causing malabsorption and diarrhea.
4. *Giardia* and cryptosporidium adhere to the surface of small bowel epithelium.

III. Approach to the Patient

A. History
   1. Time of Onset of Diarrhea.
      a. Relation to a specific meal, travel, antibiotic ingestion.
      b. Example: Staphylococcal diarrhea has very rapid (within hours) onset after ingesting foods with cream filling, salad dressings, or potato salads.
      c. Protracted diarrhea (>3 weeks) is usually due to giardiasis, amebiasis, or a noninfectious etiology.
   2. Presence of Gross Blood in the Stool.
      a. If present, bespeaks invasive agents or idiopathic colitis.
      b. If absent, suggests secretory agents, Crohn's disease, or malabsorptive syndromes.
   3. Vomiting is most common in *S. aureus* food poisoning and viral infections.
   4. Pain.
      a. Tenesmus is more common in invasive diarrhea.
      b. Right lower quadrant localization may occur in *Campylobacter* or *Yersinia* infestation.
   5. Extraintestinal Manifestation.
      a. More common in invasive diarrheas.
      b. Headaches, malaise, dizziness, and myalgias are often seen in *Campylobacter* enteropathy.
      c. Cranial neuropathy (dysarthria, diplopia, dysphagia, and mydriasis) may accompany *Clostridium botulinum* enteropathy.
   6. Travel.
      a. Diarrhea usually develops several days into the trip, but it may occur after returning home (sometimes due to lowering one's guard on the flight home).

      b. Toxigenic *E. coli* is most common, but other causes include *Shigella, Salmonella, Amoeba,* and *Giardia.*
7. Prior antibiotics (sometimes several weeks earlier).
      a. *Clostridium difficile* toxin.
8. Immunocompromised host (see below).

B. Physical Examination
1. Fever and a toxic appearance are more common in diarrheas due to invasive agents.
2. Dehydration is more common in diarrheas due to secretory agents.

C. Laboratory Data
1. Microscopic study of a fresh stool specimen (stained with methylene blue or Gram's stain).
      a. Fecal leukocytes suggest invasive diarrhea (or inflammatory bowel disease).
      b. Amebic trophozoites are best found by examining scrapings from the mucosal surface of the colon. (If invasive amebiasis or liver abscess is suspected, serologic tests such as indirect hemagglutination or gel diffusion may be necessary.)
      c. *Giardia* may not be detected because of its predilection for the upper GI tract. Diagnosis may require duodenal aspiration.
2. Stool Culture.
      a. *Campylobacter* requires specialized culture medium and incubation at 42°C, with decreased oxygen and supplemented carbon dioxide.
      b. To be considered pathogenic, *E. coli* must be serotyped or shown to produce a cytotoxin in tissue culture.
      c. If there is a history (even somewhat remote) of antibiotic ingestion, stool should be assayed for *C. difficile* toxin.

D. Sigmoidoscopy
1. Acute active colitis may be seen in *Shigella, Salmonella, Campylobacter,* and *Amoeba* infestation as well as in idiopathic ulcerative colitis.
2. Pseudomembrane formation may be seen in *C. difficile* (although the lower colon may occasionally be spared).

IV. Treatment

A. General Measures

1. Maintenance of fluid and electrolyte balance is of paramount importance.
2. Antidiarrheal agents are often prescribed before specific diagnosis is made. In most instances, this is not detrimental to the patient and does not prolong illness (exception: *Salmonella*). Useful antidiarrheal agents include bismuth subsalicylate, 60 ml or 2 tablets q.i.d.; loperamide, 2-mg capsule t.i.d.; or diphenoxylate, 1–2 2.5-mg tablets every 4 hours.
3. For virus-induced diarrhea, these are the only measures necessary or available.

B. Specific Therapies
1. *Staphylococcus Aureus.* No treatment is required, since disease is self-limited within 12–24 hours.
2. Toxigenic *Escherichia coli.*
   a. No treatment may be necessary, since the illness runs its course within several days.
   b. Trimethoprim-sulfamethoxazole, 1 double-strength tablet b.i.d., for 3–5 days shortens the duration of the illness.
   c. Doxycycline can be used for prophylaxis, as can bismuth subsalicylate.
3. *Vibrio Cholerae.*
   a. Supportive fluids and electrolytes are crucial.
   b. Tetracycline or chloramphenicol may shorten the duration of the illness.
4. *Clostridium Botulinum.*
   a. Polyvalent antitoxin, *and*
   b. Penicillin, *and*
   c. Colonic lavage.
5. *Clostridium Perfringens.* No treatment required; disease lasts less than 24 hours.
6. *Vibrio Parahemolyticus.*
   a. None, or
   b. Tetracycline.
7. *B. Cereus.* None; resolves within 12–24 hours.
8. *Shigella.*
   a. Usually none necessary due to short course of illness.
   b. In severe infection, ampicillin, 0.5–1 gram/day or trimethoprim-sulfamethoxazole.
9. *Salmonella.*

    a. Usually no treatment necessary or indicated.
    b. Treatment may be indicated in immunocompromised, debilitated patients or those with artificial prosthesis or typhoid fever.
    c. Ampicillin, chloramphenicol, amoxicillin, or trimethoprim-sulfamethoxazole, depending upon organisms' sensitivity.
    d. N.B.: Long-term carriers of *Salmonella* should be investigated for gallstones.
  10. *Campylobacter.*
    a. No treatment in mild cases, or
    b. Erythromycin, 500 mg q.i.d. for 5 days.
  11. *C. Difficile.*
    a. Withdrawal of implicated antibiotics.
    b. Metronidazole, 250 mg orally, t.i.d. for 7–10 days, *or*
    c. Vancomycin, 125–500 mg orally, q.i.d. for 7–10 days.
  12. Giardiasis.
    a. Metronidazole, 250 mg orally, t.i.d. for 5–7 days, *or*
    b. Quinacrine 100 mg orally, t.i.d. for 5 days.
  13. Amebiasis.
    a. Metronidazole, 750 mg orally, t.i.d. for 5–10 days in patients who are mildly symptomatic.

ACQUIRED IMMUNE DEFICIENCY SYNDROME (AIDS) AND THE GI TRACT

I. Clinical Considerations

A. Predisposing Cause
The immune defect in patients with AIDS (a deficiency in helper/inducer T lymphocyte-mediated immune response) predisposes them to many infections of the GI tract. Isolated organisms may be nonpathogenic in immunocompetent hosts.
B. Etiology Often Elusive
Often, a specific cause cannot be found for GI symptoms in these patients (AIDS enteropathy).
C. Cause and Effect Often Uncertain
Unfortunately, there is often a poor correlation between cul-

tures, biopsies, and the patient's clinical state. Thus, a positive culture or biopsy may not establish the cause for the patient's symptoms.

D. Refractory Treatment

Because of the underlying defect in AIDS patients, many infections are not easily eradicated by treatment and tend to recur when treatment is completed.

E. Presenting Complaints

GI-related symptoms encountered in AIDS patients include: weight loss, dysphagia, odynophagia, abdominal pain, diarrhea, and rectal bleeding.

F. Pathologic Causes

These symptoms arise from coexistent infections, neoplasia, or functional impairment of the GI tract.

II. AIDS-Related Gastrointestinal Infections

A. *Candida* Esophagitis
 1. Reported in 60% of patients with AIDS.
 2. May precede other clinical features of AIDS.
 3. Symptoms: dysphagia, odynophagia, or no symptoms.
 4. Diagnosed by inspection of oral cavity for greyish-white exudate or by esophagoscopy with brushings of esophageal mucosa looking for pseudohyphae.
 5. Treatment: Mycostatin, ketoconazole, or low-dose amphotericin.
 6. High incidence of recurrence after treatment.
B. Cytomegalovirus (CMV)
 1. May be isolated from many sites in AIDS patients, especially small bowel and colon.
 2. Can lead to severe diarrhea and malabsorption.
 3. Can cause ulcerations in the GI tract, usually the colon, with occasional perforation.
 4. Diagnosis is made by biopsy, revealing large round, dense eosinophilic intranuclear inclusions.
 5. Treatment may be possible with a new derivative of acyclovir, 9-(1,3-dihydroxy-2-propoxymethyl) guanine.
C. Herpes Simplex
 1. Less commonly encountered than CMV.

2. May infect oral pharynx, esophagus, rectum, and perianal area.
3. Ulcerations may be large, hemorrhagic, and necrotic.
4. Diagnosis can be made by seeing multinucleated giant cells in scrapings from lesions.
5. Treatment: acyclovir.

D. Cryptosporidiosis
1. A parasitic protozoan.
2. Can produce profuse, watery, cholera-like diarrhea.
3. Diagnosis either by intestinal biopsy, revealing 2- to 5-micron spheres adherent to microvilli, or by seeing oocytes in stool that is Giemsa or acid-fast stained.

E. *Mycobacterium Avium-Intracellulare*
1. Normally an environmental saprophyte.
2. Can produce colitis or small bowel enteritis in AIDS patients.
3. Diagnosis by acid-fast stain or growth in selected culture.
4. Combination antituberculous chemotherapy can be tried, but there is often resistance.

F. *Salmonella*
Especially *Salmonella typhimurium* with bacteremia (see IV, above).

G. *Campylobacter, Amoeba,* and *Giardia*
See IV, above.

III. AIDS-Related Gastrointestinal Neoplasm

A. Kaposi's Sarcoma
1. Fifty to eighty percent of AIDS patients with Kaposi's sarcoma will have GI involvement.
2. Duodenum and rectum are the most common sites.
3. Barium studies may reveal nodular lesions that are indistinguishable from lymphoma.
4. Endoscopy demonstrates characteristic red-purple nodules that are often negative on biopsy due to submucosal tumor.

B. Non-Hodgkin's Lymphoma
Intraorally, rectally, or in the small bowel.

C. Cloacogenic Carcinoma

D. Squamous Carcinoma
  1. Tongue.
  2. Anorectal.

SUGGESTED READINGS

Dickinson GM: Gastrointestinal infections in patients with human immunodeficiency virus infection. *Curr Concepts Gastroenterol* 13:3–8, 1989.

Gelb A, Miller S: AIDS and gastroenterology. *Am J Gastroenterol* 81: 619–622, 1986.

Smith PD: Gastrointestinal infection in patients with acquired immunodeficiency syndrome. *Viewpoints Dig Dis* 18:1–4, 1986.

Chapter 13

Inflammatory Bowel Disease

Jacob S. Walfish, M.D.
David B. Sachar, M.D.

I. Definition

The term *chronic idiopathic inflammatory bowel disease* (IBD) encompasses ulcerative colitis and Crohn's disease. *Ulcerative colitis* is a diffuse mucosal inflammation that affects the rectum and either all or part of the contiguous large intestine. *Crohn's disease* is a transmural inflammation that can involve any segment of the alimentary tract from mouth to anus. The ileum alone is involved (ileitis) in about 30–35% of cases, both ileum and (usually adjacent) colon (ileocolitis) in about 45%, and colon alone (Crohn's colitis) in about 20%; rarely, the predominant involvement is in other areas such as stomach, duodenum, esophagus, or appendix. Although many clinical and epidemiologic features may overlap, at least 90% of cases of IBD can be classified as either ulcerative colitis or Crohn's disease.

II. Etiology

A. Infectious Agents

Infectious agents are prime suspects, especially mycobacteria in Crohn's disease, although their specificity and etiologic role are still unproven.

B. Immunologic Factors

Immunologic factors are widely implicated, especially disordered immunoregulatory mechanisms, although their primary pathogenetic role is also still controversial.

C. Genetic Influences

Genetic influences are strongly suspected on the basis of unequivocal familial tendencies and certain ethnic and racial predilections, but the relative contributions of heredity and environment have not been fully sorted out.

D. Psychosomatic Factors

Psychosomatic origins were postulated in past decades, but most current evidence refutes this hypothesis; confusion with so-called "spastic colitis" or "mucous colitis" (obsolete misnomers for irritable bowel syndrome) has contributed to the persisting misconception of inflammatory bowel diseases as primarily emotional disorders.

III. Clinical Features

A. Ulcerative Colitis

1. *Bloody diarrhea* is the hallmark.

   a. Formed stools mixed with blood and mucus suggest limited distal disease (proctitis or proctosigmoiditis); urgency is common, but diffuse abdominal pain and constitutional symptoms are rare in this form of the disease.

   b. Looser and more copious stools, often associated with abdominal pain and tenderness, weight loss, fever, and/or anemia, indicate more extensive colitis.

2. Extracolonic Manifestations.

   a. Joints.

      i. Peripheral arthritis, usually associated with activity of bowel disease.

      ii. Ankylosing spondylitis and sacroiliitis, independent of colitis activity but associated with HLA haplotype B27.

   b. Skin.

      i. Erythema nodosum, usually associated with colitis activity.

      ii. Pyoderma gangrenosum, associated with clinical activity of the colitis in about half the cases, but sometimes apparently independent.

   c. Eyes.

      i. Episcleritis or keratoconjunctivitis, usually associated with colitis activity.

      ii. Anterior uveitis, independent of colitis activity but, like spondylitis and sacroiliitis, associated with HLA-B27.

   d. Biliary Tree.

      i. Sclerosing cholangitis may complicate cases of young onset, even after colectomy.

      ii. Bile duct cancer is an occasional late complication, with a history of ulcerative colitis occurring in approximately half the western world's cases of cholangiocarcinoma.

B. Crohn's Disease

  1. Chronic Inflammation.

   a. The most frequent presentation.

   b. Produces diarrhea, abdominal pain, fever, tender right lower quadrant fullness or mass.

  2. Intestinal Obstruction.

   a. Results from combinations of spasm, edema, and fibrotic stenosis.

   b. A very frequent late manifestation; occasionally the initial presentation.

  3. Diffuse Jejunoileitis.

   a. A combined picture of inflammation and obstruction.

   b. Results in chronic disability and malnutrition.

  4. Fistulization. Deep sinus tracts and transmural inflammation frequently penetrate the bowel wall and burrow into adjacent structures to produce:

   a. Mesenteric sinuses and intramesenteric abscesses.

   b. Enteroenteric fistulae.

   c. Enterovesical fistulae (often manifested by dysuria, pneumaturia, and recurrent infection).

   d. Retroperitoneal fistulae with psoas abscess and noncalculous hydroureter and hydronephrosis (often manifested by pain in the hip, thigh, or knee, with an associated limp).

  e. Enterocutaneous fistulae (sometimes emerging from the umbilicus, flank, or groin, but most commonly presenting through the site of a previous surgical scar).

 5. Perianal Fistulae and Abscesses.

  a. Infection spreads from anal crypts of Morgagni into intersphincteric spaces.

  b. Occur in about one-third of patients, independent of activity or severity of intraabdominal disease.

  c. Often the earliest sign of Crohn's disease; rarely the sole manifestation.

 6. Extraintestinal Manifestations.

  a. Comprise the same joint, skin, eye, and perhaps biliary complications seen in ulcerative colitis.

  b. Aphthous stomatitis.

  c. Amyloidosis in cases of long-standing inflammation and/or suppuration.

IV. Diagnosis and Differential Diagnosis

 A. Ulcerative Colitis

  1. *Sigmoidoscopy* is the key to prompt initial diagnosis. A simple rigid sigmoidoscope examination is usually adequate to reveal the characteristic friability, granularity, scattered hemorrhages, and loss of normal mucosal vascular pattern; more severe cases might manifest gross mucosal ulcerations with purulent exudate. Total colonoscopy is *not* indicated and invites a risk of perforation in acute cases.

  2. *Plain films* of the abdomen may be helpful in judging the extent and severity of the colitis by showing accumulation of gas in paralyzed or even dilated segments of colon, loss of haustration, submucosal edema, and/or absence of formed stool in the diseased bowel. Barium enema is *not* indicated and entails a risk of perforation in acute cases.

  3. *Microbiologic studies* to rule out infectious colitis are absolutely mandatory. Stool cultures, microscopic examination, toxin assays, and blood serology are essential in differentiating ulcerative colitis from infectious colitis due to *Salmonella, Shigella, Campylobacter,* amebiasis, gonorrhea, syphilis, herpes, *Chlamydia,* cytomegalovirus (CMV), or *Clostridium difficile.*

4. *Rectal biopsy* may be of value in occasionally establishing a specific infectious etiology, or at least in distinguishing an acute self-limited colitis (ASLC) from chronic idiopathic IBD. Distortion of crypt architecture, separation of crypts, and infiltration of the lamina propria by chronic mononuclear inflammatory cells characterize chronic IBD as opposed to ASLC.

5. *Other specific colitides* include those related to ischemia; radiation; and oral contraceptives, antibiotics, or other drugs and toxins.

B. Crohn's Disease

1. *Small bowel x-rays* with spot films of the terminal ileum will readily establish the diagnosis in most cases of ileitis. Irregularity, nodularity, deep ulcers or sinus tracts, cobblestoning, narrowing, pseudodiverticulosis, and separation of loops are characteristic features. The diagnosis is likely to be missed, however, if one routinely orders an "upper GI series" without specifically requesting small bowel follow-through and compression spot films of the terminal ileum.

2. *Appendicitis* is the most common differential diagnosis in cases with acute presentation of right lower quadrant pain, tenderness, and inflammatory signs, but a careful history will usually elicit additional symptoms such as chronic pain, diarrhea, anorexia, malaise, weight loss, fevers, or anemia in patients with Crohn's disease.

3. *Acute terminal ileitis* is an acute self-limited infection, usually due to *Yersinia enterocolitica*, generally distinguished by its acute course, and best diagnosed by specific stool cultures and serology.

4. *Other diseases* mimicking ileitis include chronic appendiceal abscess, tubo-ovarian disease, ileocecal tuberculosis, amebiasis, vasculitis, and primary or metastatic small bowel neoplasms.

C. Crohn's versus Ulcerative Colitis

At least 95% of cases of Crohn's disease of the colon can be distinguished from ulcerative colitis by one or more of the following features:

1. Small bowel involvement.

2. Rectal sparing.

3. Absence of rectal bleeding.

4. Segmental or asymmetrical distribution.
5. Perianal disease.
6. Associated mass or fistulae.
7. Patchy lesions or aphthoid, longitudinal, or serpiginous ulceration on endoscopy.
8. Transmural disease or granulomas on biopsy.

V. Complications

A. Ulcerative Colitis
1. Massive Hemorrhage. An infrequent complication, but one that usually requires urgent colectomy.
2. Toxic Fulminant Colitis. A syndrome that is due to deep transmural dissection of the ulcerating inflammatory process, resulting in lcoalized peritoneal signs (silent, painful, tender abdomen), systemic toxicity (fever, tachycardia, leukocytosis), and at least segmental and sometimes more generalized paralysis of bowel motility (abdominal distention, decreased bowel frequency). A late consequence may be so-called *toxic dilatation* (*"megacolon"*), but it is essential to recognize and treat toxic colitis *before* this late complication of colonic dilatation develops.
3. Colorectal Cancer. After the first 10 years of chronic ulcerative colitis, irrespective of the age at onset or the clinical severity of the disease, there is an approximately 0.5–1% annual incidence of colorectal cancer; this cancer risk is at least 20-fold higher than the risk in a standard age- and sex-matched population, and it rises progressively as the anatomic extent of the colitis increases from left-sided to universal. A preclinical warning sign of impending malignant change is cellular atypia or *dysplasia* on colonic mucosal biopsy, especially in conjunction with a grossly visible mass lesion or elevation in the mucosa; it is therefore becoming common practice to conduct routine colonoscopic surveillance of ulcerative colitis patients every year or two after their first 8–10 years of disease, although the actual cost-benefit ratios of various surveillance regimens have not been definitively established.

B. Crohn's disease
1. Malabsorption due to:

    a. Very extensive small bowel disease or resection (>80 cm).
    b. Bacterial overgrowth secondary to stricturing and/or fistulization.
    c. "Short-circuiting" caused by fistulization.
2. Renal Disease.
    a. Kidney Stones.
       i Uric acid due to increased metabolism and/or impaired urinary dilution and alkalinization.
      ii. Calcium oxalate due to increased colonic oxalate absorption ("enteric hyperoxaluria").
    b. Urinary infections, especially with bladder fistulae.
    c. Hydroureter and hydronephrosis (see III.B.4.d).
    d. Amyloidosis (see III.B.6.c).
3. Gallstones. Due to impaired bile salt reabsorption from terminal ileum.
4. Cancer.
    a. Increased risk of both small and large bowel cancer.
    b. Associated with very long-standing disease.

VI. Medical Management of Ulcerative Colitis

A. Mild or Limited Colitis
  1. Symptomatic Therapy.
    a. Diet.
       i. Low-roughage diet may be helpful.
      ii. Elimination of milk may ameliorate symptoms in about one-third of patients but need not be continued if no benefit is noted.
    b. Antidiarrheal Agents.
       i. Useful for mild to moderate cases, but contraindicated in severe or toxic cases so as to avoid precipitating toxic dilatation.
      ii. Regimens include diphenoxylate 2.5–5 mg, loperamide 2–4 mg, deodorized tincture of opium (DTO) 10–15 drops, or codeine 15–30 mg, two to four times a day as required.
    c. Bulk Formers.
       i. Example: psyllium hydrophilic mucilloid.
      ii. May alleviate complaints of frequent scanty rectal discharges with tenesmus.

    iii. Use with more fluid for hard, pellet-like stools and with less fluid for loose or watery discharges.

2. *Rectal instillations* (indicated for limited proctosigmoiditis or for predominant symptoms of tenesmus).

    a. Steroids.

        i. Hydrocortisone enemas (100 mg in 60 ml) most convenient at night; may reach as far as splenic flexure if hips elevated.

        ii. Hydrocortisone foam (10%) or suppositories (25 mg) more convenient in daytime; tend to concentrate effects in rectum.

    b. 5-Aminosalicylic acid (5-ASA) (4 grams in 60 ml); often effective in refractory cases.

3. *Sulfasalazine* (an azo dimer of sulfapyridine and 5-aminosalicylic acid).

    a. Indications.

        i. Mild-to-moderate colitis.

        ii. Maintenance of remission.

    b. Dosage.

        i. One-half to 1.5 gram, two to four times a day.

        ii. Introduced gradually and administered with meals.

    c. Side effects.

        i. Allergic reaction (rash, fever, arthritis): usually manageable by "desensitization" regimen, starting with 10–60 mg/day and gradually increasing the dose over several weeks.

        ii. Common symptoms (nausea, vomiting, anorexia, dyspepsia, headache): dose-related, reversible, sometimes lessened with use of enteric-coated preparations.

        iii. Mild hematologic effects (low-grade hemolysis, mild leukopenia, folate depletion and/or malabsorption): dose-related, usually controllable with folic acid supplementation.

        iv. Severe toxic reactions (alveolitis, hepatitis, pancreatitis, epidermal necrolysis, massive hemolysis, agranulocytosis): very rare, absolute contraindications to any further use at any dose.

        v. Male infertility (decreased sperm count, motility, penetrating ability; altered morphology): reversible within 1–2 months of stopping drug; not associated with teratogenicity.

    d. Use in Pregnancy.
       i. Safe throughout all of pregnancy and breast-feeding.
      ii. No increased risk of fetal abnormalities or kernicterus.
    e. Analogues.
       i. Ninety percent of adverse side effects attributable to sulfapyridine moiety of molecule.
      ii. New formulations have been developed of non-sulfa-containing 5-ASA, which have topical therapeutic action within bowel lumen.
     iii. Four hundred milligrams of monomeric 5-ASA (mesalazine) or 500 mg of dimeric 5-ASA (olsalazine) is therapeutically equivalent to 1.0 gram of sulfasalazine.

B. Moderate Colitis (Ambulatory)
  1. Oral Steroids.
    a. Prompt remission should be sought by initiating therapy at relatively high daily doses, i.e., 30–40 mg of prednisone or equivalent.
    b. Should gradually be tapered after remission is achieved, and should not be relied upon in high doses for long-term maintenance.
  2. Immunosuppressives.
    a. Antimetabolites (azathioprine or 6-mercaptopurine) are occasionally used for refractory steroid-dependent cases that are not suitable for surgery.

C. Severe Colitis (Hospitalized)
  1. Parenteral Corticoids.
    a. Intravenous Hydrocortisone.
       i. Used for patients who have recently been receiving steroid therapy.
      ii. Optimal dose approximately 300 mg per day (continuous 24-hour infusion, or else divided doses via bolus drip every 6–8 hours).
    b. Intravenous adrenocorticotropic hormone (ACTH).
       i. Might be preferable for patients who have not had recent steroid therapy.
      ii. Optimal dose approximately 120 units per day (continuous 24-hour infusion, or else divided doses via bolus drip every 6–8 hours).

    c. Duration of Therapy.
        i. Optimal duration of intravenous corticoid therapy is 7–10 days.
        ii. Cases unresponsive by 7–10 days rarely, if ever, respond to more prolonged courses, and surgery should be considered.
    d. Electrolytes.
        i. Provide supplementary potassium chloride (KCl) in intravenous fluids at approximately 20–40 mEq/L.
        ii. Do not use any intravenous sodium chloride (NaCl) except in dehydrated patients, so as to minimize steroid-induced edema.
    2. Intravenous hyperalimentation (total parenteral nutrition (TPN)) is of no primary benefit in management of ulcerative colitis.
D. Toxic (Fulminant) Colitis
   Toxic fulminant colitis with or without dilatation or "megacolon" (see V.A.2, above):
    1. Discontinue antidiarrheal drugs.
    2. Make patients NPO and pass long tube attached to intermittent suction to decompress the bowel.
    3. Give aggressive supportive care with intravenous fluids, electrolytes, and blood as indicated.
    4. Institute intravenous hydrocortisone or ACTH as outlined in VI.C.1, above.
    5. Administer intravenous broad-spectrum antibiotics.
    6. Rotate patient to prone position every few hours to redistribute colonic gas.
    7. Observe closely for signs of progressive peritonitis or even silent perforation (e.g., loss of hepatic dullness on physical examination).
    8. Obtain abdominal x-rays every day or two to monitor course of colonic dilatation and to detect free air.
    9. Follow patient with a surgeon and plan urgent colectomy within a day or two unless sustained improvement can be demonstrated unequivocally.

VII. **Surgical Management of Ulcerative Colitis**

A. Indications.
    1. Emergency

      a. Exsanguinating hemorrhage.

      b. Toxicity and/or perforation.

   2. Elective.

      a. Dysplasia or cancer.

      b. Growth retardation or other systemic complications.

      c. Intractability.

B. Procedures.

   1. Emergency. Subtotal colectomy and ileostomy with rectum maintained as mucous fistula or Hartmann pouch.

   2. Elective.

      a. Total proctocolectomy with abdominoperineal resection of rectum, and

         i. Standard (Brooke) ileostomy: incontinent, requires external appliance.

        ii. Continent ileostomy (Koch pouch): no external appliance, emptied by catheterization through nipple valve. Potential complications include valve malfunction and "pouchitis" (mucosal inflammation of pouch).

      b. Subtotal colectomy with preservation of rectum by:

         i. Simple ileorectal anastomosis: requires continual observation and often treatment of inflamed rectal mucosa.

        ii. Mucosal proctectomy ("stripping" of rectal mucosa) and ileoanal anastomosis of ileal reservoir (pelvic pouch) through sleeve of rectal sphincter muscles: potential complications include anastomotic leak and stricture, "pouchitis," and partial incontinence.

VIII. Medical Management of Crohn's Disease

A. Symptomatic Therapy
The general principles of therapy are the same as for ulcerative colitis.

B. Sulfasalazine

   1. The general principles of therapy are the same as for ulcerative colitis.

   2. Somewhat more efficacy in colonic than in pure small bowel disease.

   3. Efficacy in maintaining remissions not proven.

C. Steroids
   1. The general principles of therapy are the same as for ulcerative colitis.
   2. Relatively contraindicated for cases complicated by fistula and abscess.
D. Immunosuppressives (Azathioprine and 6-Mercaptopurine)
   1. Indications.
      a. Steroid sparing.
      b. Fistula healing.
      c. Perineal disease.
   2. Dosage.
      a. Initiated at 1.0–1.5 mg/kg; may be increased gradually up to 2.5 mg/kg.
      b. Usually requires 3–4 months before initial manifestations of therapeutic benefit are seen.
   3. Toxicity.
      a. Fever and/or Rash. Frequency about 3%, occurs early in treatment course; idiosyncratic; contraindication to rechallenge.
      b. Pancreatitis. Frequency about 2%; occurs early in treatment course; idiosyncratic; absolute contraindication to rechallenge.
      c. Drug Hepatitis. An infrequent complication, may occur very late in treatment course.
      d. Bone Marrow Depression. Dose-related; avoidance requires regular monitoring of blood counts at least monthly.
   4. Theoretical risks (susceptibility to infection, neoplasm and teratogenicity) must be considered but have not been substantiated by experience.
E. Metronidazole
   1. Indications.
      a. Perineal lesions.
      b. Mild to moderate colitis, ileocolitis, and perhaps ileitis.
   2. Dosage.
      a. Ranges from 10 to 30 mg/kg/day (usually 15–20 mg/kg/day) in three or four divided doses.
      b. May require several weeks before benefits are seen.
   3. Toxicity.
      a. Nausea, vomiting, anorexia: dose-related.
      b. Altered taste, furry tongue: dose-related.

       c. Peripheral neuropathy: dose-related, frequency 30–50%; usually reversible, but often obviates continued use.

F. Other Antibiotics
    1. Clearly useful in managing suppurative complications of fistula and abscess.
    2. Widespread anecdotal experience of benefit when used as primary therapy, despite absence of controlled clinical trials.

G. Enteral and Parenteral Hyperalimentation
Defined and elemental diets, TPN.
    1. As Adjunctive Therapy.
       a. Nutritional repletion, especially preoperatively, in malnourished patients.
       b. Induction of growth spurts in children with growth failure.
       c. Promotion of fistula healing.
       d. Alleviation of chronic obstructive symptoms.
       e. Maintenance of nutrition in short-bowel syndrome.
    2. As Primary Therapy. Role in possible long-term improvement of natural history of disease is still under study.

IX. Surgical Management of Crohn's Disease

A. Frequency
Approximately 70% of patients with Crohn's disease ultimately require surgery.

B. Indications
    1. Specific Complications.
       a. Chronic obstruction.
       b. Abscess.
       c. Complicated fistulae if they are symptomatic, producing obstruction or infection, and unresponsive to antibiotics, immunosuppressives, and enteral or parenteral regimens of bowel rest.
       d. Perforation.
       e. Massive bleeding.
    2. Chronic debility ("medical intractability").

C. Procedures
    1. Conventional. Resection of grossly diseased segments of bowel, with closure of fistulas and maximal preservation of normal intestine.

2. "Conservative." The newer and relatively experimental approach of dilating strictures ("strictureplasty") is being applied to areas of stenotic obstruction when the lesions are too extensive to permit resection. The latter approach is still favored whenever feasible.

D. Postoperative Recurrence
1. *Symptomatic recurrence,* almost always occurring at the site of anastomosis, appears at a relatively constant rate of approximately 10% per year.
2. *Reoperation* is ultimately required in approximately 40–50% of all patients after first resection, and in about 25% of those patients who have undergone two operations. Among all Crohn's disease patients, therefore, approximately 70% undergo one operation, 30% undergo two operations, and only about 8% undergo three or more operations.
3. *Prevention of recurrence* is a desideratum that no postoperative prophylactic regimen has ever been shown to achieve.
4. *Psychosocial rehabilitation,* on the other hand, is successfully accomplished in about 80% of all patients who undergo surgery, so that operations should not be withheld when the indications are clear.

SUGGESTED READINGS

Bayless TM (ed): *Current Management of Inflammatory Bowel Disease.* Philadelphia, BC Decker, 1989.

Kirsner JB, Shorter RD (eds): *Inflammatory Bowel Disease,* ed 3. Philadelphia, Lea & Febiger, 1988.

Chapter 14

Vascular Disorders of the Intestine

Blair S. Lewis, M.D.

I. Normal Circulation

A. Arterial Supply
  1. Celiac Axis (Fig. 14.1).
     a. Supplies the spleen, liver, pancreas, stomach, and duodenum.
     b. Branches.
        i. The splenic artery supplies the greater curvature of the stomach through the short gastric artery and the left gastroepiploic artery.
        ii. The left gastric artery supplies the lesser curvature of the stomach.
        iii. The hepatic artery also supplies the stomach and pancreas through the gastroduodenal artery, which has two branches: the right gastroepiploic artery and the superior pancreaticoduodenal artery.
     c. With such a varied blood supply, the stomach is not prone to ischemia.
  2. Superior Mesenteric Artery (SMA) (Fig. 14.2).
     a. Supplies the pancreas, duodenum, jejunum, ileum, cecum, and the portion of the colon from the right colon to the midtransverse colon.
     b. Branches.
        i. The jejunal branches supply the jejunum and ileum.

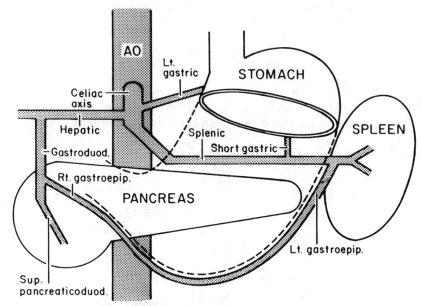

Figure 14.1. Celiac axis.

    ii. The interior pancreaticoduodenal artery supplies the pancreas and duodenum.

    iii. The middle colic artery supplies the proximal transverse colon.

    iv. The right colic artery supplies the ascending colon and hepatic flexure.

    v. The ileocolic artery supplies the jejunum, ileum, cecum, and ascending colon.

   c. The SMA is a large vessel with an angled takeoff from the aorta, making it the major site for embolization. Ninety-five percent of mesenteric emboli originating from the heart lodge in the SMA or one of its branches.

   d. The jejunal and ileal arteries form three or four arcades and enter the small bowel wall as end arteries called arteriae rectae. Occlusion of these end arteries leads to segmental infarction.

3. Inferior Mesenteric Artery (IMA) (Fig. 14.3).

   a. Supplies the distal transverse colon, descending colon, sigmoid, and proximal rectum.
   b. Branches.
      i. Left colic artery.
      ii. Sigmoid artery.
      iii. Superior rectal artery.
   c. Smallest caliber of the aortic branch arteries.
   d. May connect with the middle colic through the arc of Riolan, also called the meandering mesenteric artery.

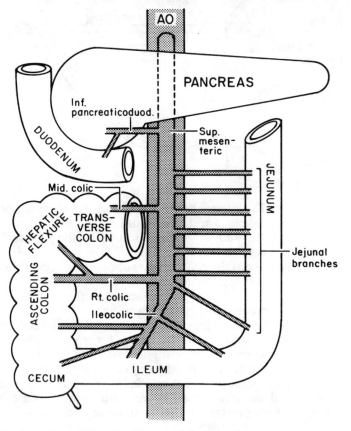

Figure 14.2. Superior mesenteric artery and its branches.

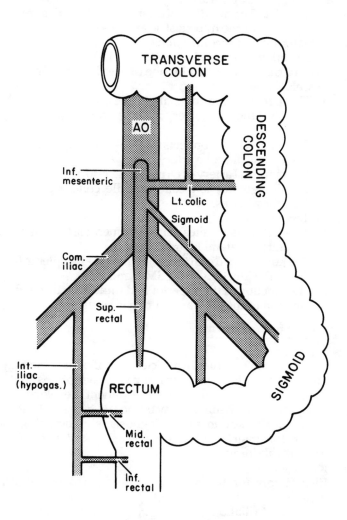

Figure 14.3. The inferior mesenteric artery and its branches.

    4. Internal Iliac Artery.
       a. Branches.
          i. Hypogastric artery.
             a. The middle and inferior rectal arteries are branches
                 of the hypogastric artery.
  B. Anastomotic Interconnections
     These allow collateral flow (Fig. 14.4). All intraabdominal
     viscera can be supplied by one of the three major mesenteric
     vessels.
     1. The pancreaticoduodenal arcades, one from the hepatic
        branch of the celiac artery and one from the MSA, supply the
        pancreas.
     2. The arc of Riolan connects the IMA's left colic artery with the
        SMA's middle colic artery.
     3. The marginal artery of Drummond is formed from branches
        of the sigmoid, left colic, middle colic, right colic, and
        ileocolic arteries.
  C. Watershed Areas
     Watershed areas are sites that are vulnerable to ischemia due to
     inadequate collateral blood supply.
     1. The junction of distal transverse colon and splenic flexure—
        this is the junction of the SMA and IMA.
     2. The junction of the superior and middle rectum—this is the
        junction of the IMA and hypogastric artery.

II. **Approach to the Patient**

  A. Introduction
     Patients with vascular insufficiency of the intestine may pres-
     ent with very few symptoms, or with symptoms that mimic
     other diseases. By the time the patient develops clear-cut
     symptoms of ischemia, it may be too late to institute life-saving
     therapy. The key to early diagnosis is recognizing the risk
     factors for small bowel ischemia in a high-risk patient present-
     ing with abdominal pain.
  B. Risk Factors
     Risk factors for the development of small bowel ischemia
     include:
     1. Atrial fibrillation.
     2. Atherosclerotic disease, e.g., stroke, angina, myocardial
        infarction, peripheral vascular disease.

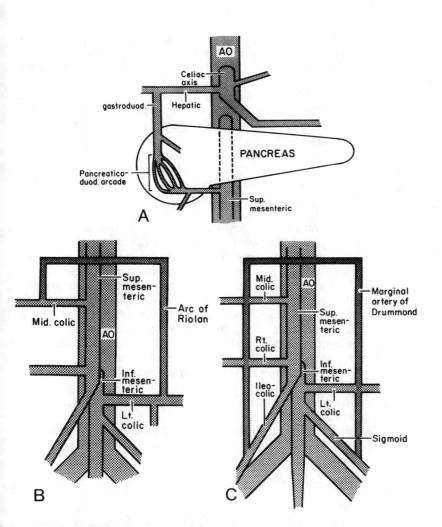

Figure 14.4. Collateral flow: A, pancreaticoduodenal arcades; B, arc of Riolan; C, marginal artery of Drummond.

    3. Low-flow states, e.g., congestive heart failure, shock.
    4. History of abdominal angina.
  C. Two Major Symptoms
    1. Pain.
      a. Although colitis or infarcted bowel classically produces localized pain with peritoneal signs, small bowel ischemia may present with midline pain and no associated physical findings.
      b. It must be stressed that, although small bowel ischemia and colonic ischemia may occasionally present similarly, they usually act very differently and have different prognoses.
    2. Bleeding. Frank bleeding is more indicative of colonic disease. Patients with small bowel ischemia may have occult blood in their stool, but they rarely present with hematochezia.
  D. Evaluation
    1. Angiography. Whenever small bowel ischemia is considered a possibility, angiography is the first order of business. Angiography requires proper interpretation, however, since many elderly patients at risk for ischemia disease have atherosclerotic disease with arterial narrowing, but are not suffering from ischemia. It is possible to supply all the visceral organs from a single aortic branch. Angiography is further complicated in these patients because those chosen for examination are usually hypotensive and vasoconstricted. Angiographic contrast increases cardiac output and flow in the injected artery. These factors make recognition and interpretation of low flow difficult.
    2. In the absence of pain, it is possible to observe the patient and consider other possibilities.
    3. Painless bleeding should be handled as any other case of hematochezia. Stabilization and observation are the key to managing lower GI hemorrhage.

III. Mesenteric Ischemia

  A. Abdominal Angina
    1. Pathophysiology. Like coronary artery disease, abdominal angina reflects an imbalance of supply and demand. Patients with fixed atherosclerotic narrowing of the splanchnic

arteries are unable to increase splanchnic blood flow to match demand during food digestion.

2. Clinical and Laboratory Features.
   a. Pain—crampy, dull, usually periumbilical pain occurring 15–30 minutes postprandially and lasting for hours. This is a warning of imminent catastrophe, since many patients go on to acute mesenteric infarction within weeks or months.
   b. Fear of eating is a classic symptom. Patients do not eat for fear of developing abdominal pain.
   c. Weight loss is a common finding. This is due to decreased food intake.
   d. Physical examination of the abdomen is usually normal, although an abdominal bruit may be heard.
   e. History and physical examination may provide evidence of other atherosclerotic disease, e.g., stroke, angina, myocardial infarction, peripheral vascular disease.
   f. Laboratory tests are normal. Fecal occult blood test is negative.
3. Diagnosis. Angiography in the patient with the above symptoms shows two of three vessels with >50% narrowing.
4. Management. Surgery with bypass grafting, reimplantation of the vessel, or endarterectomy.

B. Acute Mesenteric Infarction
   1. Pathophysiology.
      a. Acute occlusion of the SMA or one of its branches. Usually occurs in the setting of atherosclerotic disease in which collateral flow is compromised.
      b. Source of the occlusion may be:
         i. Thrombotic occlusion of an already narrowed atherosclerotic lesion.
         ii. Embolism, usually from the heart in a patient with arrhythmia or valvular disease.
         iii. Obstruction secondary to an aortic dissection or vasculitis.
      c. Responsible for 75% of cases of small bowel ischemia.
      d. Carries an 80% mortality.
   2. Clinical and Laboratory Features.
      a. Patients present with the acute onset of severe periumbilical abdominal pain. The pain is out of proportion to

findings on physical and laboratory exam. Fifty percent of patients give a history of abdominal angina. At this time, physical exam can be normal, with a negative fecal occult blood test.

b. Without early intervention, symptoms progress and the patient develops frank peritonitis with fever, leukocytosis, and eventually shock, sepsis, and death.

c. Severe, uncorrectable, metabolic acidosis without another source is a hallmark of intestinal infarction.

3. Management.

a. Initial evaluation following supportive care with intravenous fluids should include a complete blood cell count (CBC) to demonstrate leukocytosis. Abdominal x-ray can show an ileus early in the course.

b. Angiography can confirm the clinical diagnosis of occlusion of the SMA or its branches.

c. Surgery is necessary for the patient's survival. Necrotic bowel must be resected. It may be difficult to visually differentiate irreversibly ischemic or dead bowel from cyanotic, yet viable, tissue. During the laparotomy, the surgeon can assess viability of tissue (a) visually; (b) by observing for peristalsis or palpating for pulses; (c) by using Doppler ultrasonography to see if there is blood flow to the area in question; or (d) by using fluorescein angiography.

d. Many centers advocate reoperation in 12–36 hours, so-called second-look surgery, to rule out extension of necrosis.

C. Nonocclusive Intestinal Infarction

1. Pathophysiology.

a. Results from poor perfusion in already compromised bowel. Fixed atherosclerotic lesions are made symptomatic by decreased blood flow and vasoconstriction.

b. Transmural infarction is most common, but sometimes the process is limited only to the mucosal layer.

c. Accounts for 15% of cases of small bowel ischemia.

2. Clinical and Laboratory Features.

a. The clinical setting is one of poor perfusion, e.g., shock (from some other cause, such as sepsis or trauma); anoxia;

congestive heart failure; recent myocardial infarction; or the use of certain medications (especially vasopressors and digitalis) that cause splanchnic vasoconstriction.
   b. Angiography shows no occlusion to flow; it shows:
      i. Narrow, irregular SMA branches.
      ii. Spasm of the arcades.
      iii. Impaired filling of intramural vessels.
   3. Management. Initial therapy includes use of continuous infusion of vasodilators (e.g., papaverine) into selected arteries.
D. Mesenteric Venous Thrombosis
   1. Pathophysiology.
      a. Occlusion of the SMV (in 95% of cases), in turn causing decreased arterial flow to the bowel.
      b. Responsible for 10% of cases of small bowel ischemia.
      c. Etiologies: portal hypertension, congestive heart failure, pancreatic cancer, peritonitis, inflammatory bowel disease, intraabdominal abscess, intraabdominal surgery or trauma, hypercoagulable states (due to causes such as polycythemia vera, antithrombin 3 deficiency, oral contraceptive pills).
   2. Clinical and Laboratory Features.
      a. Seventy percent of patients present with a 2- to 3-day history of abdominal pain and diarrhea. Pain slowly increases in severity. Nausea and vomiting often develop.
      b. Initially, physical exam can be normal except for a positive fecal occult blood test. Without intervention, infarction and signs of peritonitis develop.

IV. **Ischemic Colitis**

   A. Pathogenesis
      1. Most commonly secondary to nonocclusive low flow to the colon, although embolic obstruction does occur. Causes include:
         a. Low-flow states such as shock, recent myocardial infarction, congestive heart failure.
         b. Operations that sacrifice the IMA or its branches, e.g., abdominal aortic aneurysm repair or abdominoperineal

resection. Since ischemic colitis occurs in 0.5–2% of these cases, preoperative angiography or intraoperative Doppler exams are often performed to assess collateral flow.

   c. Less commonly, amyloidosis, vasculitis, hypercoagulable states, and use of oral contraceptive pills.

2. The most common sites of involvement are the watershed areas where there is least collateral blood flow, viz., the points where the distal transverse colon meets the splenic flexure and where the superior rectum meets the middle rectum. The lower rectum is usually spared in ischemic colitis except in patients who have had aortic aneurysm repair.

3. In 20% of cases, there is a predisposing obstructive colonic lesion distal to the ischemic area. These lesions include cancer, diverticulitis, colonic stricture, or Hirschsprung's disease.

B. Clinical Features

1. Ischemic colitis can present in a spectrum of severity ranging from self-limited, segmental disease that heals within 4 weeks, to fulminant colitis that progresses to necrosis and perforation.

2. Ninety percent of patients present with self-limited, segmental colitis. Painless rectal bleeding is the most common presenting symptom. Plain abdominal x-ray or barium enema shows "thumb-printing," which represents intramural hemorrhage and edema. There is no specific therapy, and most cases resolve without incident. A few patients can go on to develop colonic strictures as a result of healing with fibrosis.

3. Patients with a more severe form of ischemic colitis present with abdominal pain and rectal bleeding. The abdominal pain is usually located over the involved area and is usually associated with abdominal tenderness on examination. Fever and leukocytosis are also indicative of a more severe process.

C. Differential Diagnosis

1. The diagnosis on presentation is usually not clear, and the differential diagnosis includes diverticulitis and perforated colonic carcinoma.

2. Ischemic colitis should not be confused with acute mesenteric ischemia, in which the pain is periumbilical and hematochezia is uncommon.

D. Management
   1. Initial management is supportive, with intravenous fluids and antibiotics. The immediate use of barium enema or colonoscopy carries substantial risk of precipitating free perforation. Use of these tests once the patient has stabilized (as evidenced by improvement of physical exam, fever, and leukocytosis) usually yields the correct diagnosis.
   2. The fulminant form of ischemic colitis may require surgical resection of the involved colon.

V. Radiation Enteritis and Colitis

A. Pathophysiology
   1. Occurs in approximately 10% of patients who have received radiation therapy for malignancy, either intestinal or extraintestinal.
   2. Site of Involvement.
      a. Esophagus. Secondary to radiation treatment of bronchial cancer, Hodgkin's lymphoma, or primary radiotherapy of esophageal cancer. The esophagus, however, is the most radioresistant organ in the GI tract, tolerating 6000–7000 rads total dose.
      b. Small Intestine and Colon. Secondary to radiation treatment of pelvic cancers, e.g., cervical, prostatic, testicular, ovarian, or rectal.
   3. Factors Determining Susceptibility to Radiation Damage.
      a. Toxicity is dose-dependent. There is a low toxic:therapeutic dose ratio.
      b. Toxic doses are measured in two ways:
         i. Minimum tolerance dose (TD/5/5) is the dose at which 1–5% of patients develop injury within 5 years. This is approximately 4000 rads total dose in the small and large bowel.
         ii. Maximum tolerance dose (TD/50/5) is the dose at which 25–50% of patients develop injury within 5 years. This is approximately 5000 rads total dose in the small and large bowel.

c. Other than total dose, there are other factors that determine susceptibility to radiation damage.
   i. Location of the radiation given (whether to stomach, esophagus, or intestine; and which intervening organs protect the bowel).
   ii. Concomitant vascular disease limiting blood flow to the radiated area and thereby increasing the likelihood of damage.
   iii. Concomitant chemotherapy that also damages actively replicating mucosa.
   iv. Previous pelvic surgery or pelvic inflammatory disease, which fixes the normally mobile small bowel into the pelvis and thus makes it more susceptible to radiation damage.
4. Acute Effects of Radiation. Mucosa, with its rapidly dividing cells, is most susceptible to radiation and shows its effects first. At high doses, there can be focal ulceration of the mucosa, necrosis, and even perforation with peritonitis.
5. Late Effects of Radiation.
   a. Submucosal arterioles are also very radiosensitive and respond to radiation with swelling and proliferation of individual endothelial cells within 2–12 months. These changes within the endothelium lead to obstruction to blood flow (obliterative endarteritis and endophlebitis) and thrombosis within the vessel.
   b. This vascular effect leads to many other manifestations of radiation disease.
      i. Neovascularization with mucosal telangiectasias.
      ii. Focal ischemia with ulceration or necrosis and perforation.
      iii. Delayed healing and fistulization.
      iv. Infection and abscess formation.
   c. Radiation also affects mesenchymal tissue, leading to fibrous bands and strictures.
B. Clinical Features
1. Early Symptoms.
   a. Occur immediately after radiation therapy, typically in a patient treated with pelvic radiation with a total dose >4000 rads. The presence of early symptoms does not

necessarily signify the development of late symptoms.
b. Proctitis with diarrhea and tenesmus may occur as a
   result of direct mucosal damage. Gross bleeding is an
   uncommon feature, though most patients will be positive
   on a fecal occult blood test.
c. Small bowel involvement is manifested acutely by periumbilical abdominal pain. Diarrhea may be a major
   symptom secondary to malabsorption of bile salts or
   development of lactose intolerance due to blunting of the
   mucosa.
2. Late Symptoms.
   a. These may occur 3 months to more than 20 years after
      radiation therapy. Many of the patients who develop late
      symptoms did not have early symptoms.
   b. Small bowel obstruction may develop secondary to stric-
      ture of a small bowel loop or secondary to diffuse perito-
      neal adhesions.
   c. Fistulas and abscesses may appear, especially rectovagi-
      nal fistulas after pelvic radiation for cervical cancer.
   d. Bleeding occurs secondary to mucosal telangiectasias.
   e. Malabsorption arises because of abnormal small bowel
      mucosa or bacterial overgrowth behind a partially ob-
      structed loop of small bowel.
C. Diagnosis
   1. In radiation proctitis, sigmoidoscopy reveals discolored,
      edematous mucosa.
   2. Evaluation of the patient with early or late symptoms can be
      carried out with barium studies or endoscopy.
D. Management
   1. Minimize intestinal damage prior to radiation therapy.
      a. Medical therapy such as aspirin to decrease
         prostaglandins.
      b. Elemental diet.
      c. At surgery prior to radiation, place a synthetic sling to
         raise the small bowel out of the pelvis.
   2. Bleeding is usually from neovascularization in the recto-
      sigmoid. Most of these patients do well without specific
      therapy. In some cases, sulfasalazine or topical steroids in
      the form of enemas may be effective. Surgical resection of the

involved area is ill-advised, since poor healing in these ischemic areas may produce stricture and/or fistula formation. Diversion of fecal stream with a diverting colostomy is also generally ineffective.

3. Obstruction, secondary to strictures or adhesions, is best treated surgically.

4. Fistulas, like bleeding, are not amenable to surgical resection because of poor healing. Diverting colostomy is treatment of choice.

5. Chronic diarrhea is secondary to bacterial overgrowth, malabsorption of bile salts, or lactose intolerance. Treatment therefore comprises antibiotics, cholestyramine, and avoidance of milk products.

VI. Arteriovenous Malformations (AVMs)

A. Pathophysiology

1. AVMs are small, submucosal collections of dilated arterial, venous, and capillary vessels that can be a source of bleeding.
   a. Multiple terms for AVMs: vascular dysplasia, angiodysplasia, or vascular ectasia.
   b. AVMs are different from hemangiomas, which are benign vascular tumors commonly found in the stomach, small bowel, and rectum.

2. Increasing incidence with increasing age. Average age of patients with AVMs is 69. Up to 50% of patients over the age of 60 will have AVMs present in their colons; most of these are asymptomatic.

3. Location.
   a. Seventy-eight percent of colonic AVMs in elderly patients are located in the cecum or right colon.
   b. AVMs are also commonly found in the stomach of patients with renal insufficiency.

4. It is unclear whether AVMs are congenital or acquired. The presently accepted theory is that AVMs represent an acquired dilatation of normal vascular structures that occurs with the degenerative changes of aging.
   a. Partial obstruction of veins coming through the muscu-

laris leads to dilatation of venules and capillaries and eventually to the loss of the precapillary sphincter.
5. There is an association of AVMs with aortic stenosis.
6. AVMs are the most common cause of recurrent lower GI hemorrhage.
B. Diagnosis
1. AVMs are small submucosal lesions and are thus not seen on barium enema.
2. Endoscopy can visualize these lesions as discrete red blushes with normal overlying mucosa. Endoscopy, however, may miss AVMs, since vasoconstriction may cause the blush to disappear.
3. Angiography with selective arterial catheterization can show an AVM in two ways. First, the tuft of dilated arterioles, capillaries, and venules can be seen. Second, the visualization of a vein during the arterial phase, a so-called "early filling vein," is also indicative of an AVM.
C. Management
1. AVMs are often an incidental finding at endoscopy of a patient without a history of bleeding. These lesions do not require therapy.
2. Endoscopic fulguration.
3. In patients with severe aortic stenosis and cecal AVMs, valve replacement may eliminate the need for specific therapy of the AVMs.
4. Surgical resection.
5. Estrogen therapy has been tried with some success in dialysis patients and patients with Rendu-Osler-Weber disease.

VII. Vasculitis of the Bowel

A. Polyarteritis Nodosa
1. Segmental necrotizing vasculitis affecting medium-sized and small arteries, including the coronary, renal, and mesenteric arteries.
2. Involvement, usually at vessel bifurcations, causes small aneurysms that may rupture or thrombose, leading to obstruction of the vessel.
3. Fifty percent of patients with polyarteritis nodosa have

mesenteric vessel involvement. These patients have abdominal pain and rectal bleeding secondary to mucosal ulceration.
4. Angiography confirms the diagnosis, and therapy with steroids is usually effective.
B. Systemic Lupus Erythematosus
1. Arteritis of small vessels yielding segmental lesions. Massive infarction rarely develops, but small vessel obstruction can cause segmental enteritis with abdominal pain, malabsorption, and in severe cases, perforation.
2. Abdominal pain occurs in 10–60% of patients with systemic lupus erythematosus. Besides mucosal ischemia, other causes include pancreatitis, serositis, or inflammation of the peritoneum.
C. Henoch-Schönlein Disease (Anaphylactoid Purpura)
1. Small vessel vasculitis secondary to immunoglobulin A deposition in the vessel wall. This is also called a hypersensitivity vasculitis. The circulating IgA immune complexes are frequently attributable either to medication or to a recent viral syndrome.
2. A classic triad seen in children and adolescents comprises palpable purpura, arthritis, and abdominal pain. Glomerulonephritis is also common. Fifty percent of affected patients develop abdominal pain with segmental ischemia. Often they present not only with pain but also with bleeding secondary to mucosal ulceration.
3. The illness is self-limited in most cases, requiring symptomatic therapy only.

SUGGESTED READINGS

Boley SJ, Sammartano R, Adams A, DiBase A, Kleinhaus S, Sprayregen S: On the nature and etiology of vascular ectasias of the colon. *Gastroenterology* 72:650–660, 1977.

Boley SJ, Schwartz SS, Williams LF Jr (ed): *Vascular Disorders of the Intestine*. New York, Appleton-Century-Crofts, 1971.

Fagin RR, Kirsner JB: Ischemic diseases of the colon. *Adv Intern Med* 17:343, 1971.

Novaks JM, Collins JT, Donowitz M, Farman J, Sheaham DG, Spiro HM: Effects of radiation on the human gastrointestinal tract. *J Clin Gastroenterol* 1:9, 1979.

Williams LF Jr: Vascular insufficiency of the intestine. *Gastroenterology* 61:757, 1971.

Chapter 15

Diverticular Disease of the Colon

Blair S. Lewis, M.D.

I. Pathophysiology and Epidemiology

   A. Overview

Diverticula of the colon are sac-like herniations of the mucosa through the muscularis propria. These are actually pseudodiverticula, since they do not include all the layers of the intestine but include only the mucosal and serosal layers. The herniations occur along the taenia coli at the sites where arteries come through the muscularis en route to the submucosa. In many patients, these herniations are associated with hypertrophy of the muscularis layer called myochosis. The sigmoid colon is the most common site of involvement (95%) of cases, with decreasing involvement proximally.

     1. The pathology of pseudodiverticula is different from that of true diverticula, which include all layers of the intestine. True diverticula are usually congenital and are not associated with myochosis. True diverticula are uncommon in the colon, except for an isolated cecal diverticulum.

     2. Diverticula of the small intestine are less common than colonic diverticula. Like colonic diverticula, most of these are pseudodiverticula occurring along the mesenteric border where blood vessels perforate and weaken the serosa and muscularis. Most small bowel diverticula occur in the

duodenum. Stasis in small bowel diverticula can be a source of bacterial overgrowth, causing malabsorption, diarrhea, and vitamin B_{12} deficiency.

   a. Meckel's diverticulum is not actually a diverticulum; rather, it is a remnant of the vitelline duct. (See Chapter 3.)

B. Frequency
Pseudodiverticula of the colon are acquired.

1. Colonic diverticulosis increases in frequency with increasing age, occurring in 20–50% of the population over age 50; there is a 5% incidence at age 50, growing to 50% by age 80.
2. Colonic diverticula are most common in Western populations and are rare in developing countries such as Nigeria.

C. Etiology
A commonly accepted hypothesis of diverticula formation holds that low-residue diets decrease the amount of intraluminal bulk, leading to muscular hypertrophy as the colon tries to move the small amount of fecal debris. Increased intraluminal pressure develops from colonic contractions of hypertrophied muscle, causing herniation of mucosa through the muscularis at the points weakened by transversing blood vessels.

1. Epidemiologic studies comparing the incidence of diverticular disease in Western countries and in African nations have suggested, but not proven, that diverticula are a direct result of refined diets.
2. The dietary theory is also supported by the finding that diverticulosis is three times more common in nonvegetarians than in vegetarians.

II. Approach to the Patient

A. Clinical Patterns
Diverticula of the colon can present in four different clinical patterns.

1. Incidental finding of diverticula on barium enema, flexible sigmoidoscopy, or colonoscopy—this is the most common presentation, occurring in the asymptomatic patient or the patient with symptoms not referable to diverticula. The term diverticulosis refers simply to the presence of diverticula. Most patients with diverticulosis remain asymptomatic.

Only 20–30% of patients with diverticula will ever develop symptoms referable to these herniations.

2. Diverticular pain—chronic abdominal pain without other pathology to explain the symptoms.
3. Diverticular bleeding.
4. Diverticulitis, occurring with the inflammation of a single diverticulum and presenting with abdominal pain and fever.

B. Differential Diagnosis

Many other diseases have symptoms similar to those of diverticular disease. It is important to have a complete differential diagnosis when evaluating a patient with colonic diverticula, since this common x-ray finding may not be the source of the patient's symptoms.

C. Examination of the Colon

Examination of the colon is made more difficult by the presence of diverticula.

1. Barium enema may easily miss intraluminal lesions such as polyps or cancer, especially in a redundant sigmoid colon with many diverticula. Moreover, inspissated barium may remain within the diverticula for days to weeks, making interpretation of other radiologic studies difficult. The risk of perforation during barium enema is increased, especially in patients with acute diverticulitis, as barium is introduced under pressure into the colon. The risk is even greater in double-contrast studies in which air is introduced under pressure.
2. Colonoscopy is made more difficult by the presence of muscular hypertrophy, strictures, and multiple orifices that confuse identification of the intestinal lumen. The possibility of pushing the instrument tip through a diverticulum increases the risk of perforation. This risk is further heightened in patients with acute diverticulitis, as well as in those in whom previous diverticulitis has produced either a stricture or tight fixation of the sigmoid.

III. **Diverticular Pain**

A. Pathogenesis

Increased muscular contractions cause increased intraluminal pressure, which produces symptoms in some patients. It seems unlikely that symptoms occur from fecal debris trapped in a diverticulum.

B. Clinical and Laboratory Features

1. Pain is the only symptom. The usual pattern is severe left lower quadrant pain without radiation, worse after meals, and relieved by bowel movements.

2. On exam, a firm, tender sigmoid loop may be felt. Rectal exam is normal, with no occult blood.

3. There is no fever or leukocytosis associated with this entity.

C. Differential Diagnosis

1. Irritable bowel syndrome—it may be difficult to differentiate this syndrome from diverticular disease. Irritable bowel is suggested in a younger patient with more diffuse symptoms. Therapy, however, is similar in both entities.

2. Colon cancer—this diagnosis should be suspected in the patient with occult fecal blood or insidious, progressive colonic obstruction.

3. Gynecologic and urologic disorders, such as pelvic inflammatory disease and ovarian cancer.

4. Colitis, including acute infections, ischemia, and idiopathic inflammatory bowel disease (ulcerative colitis and Crohn's disease).

D. Management

1. Initial evaluation of any patient with abdominal pain should include a complete history and physical exam, including pelvic and rectal examination. Depending on the degree of suspicion for other diagnoses, further testing with sigmoidoscopy and barium enema can be performed.

2. Diet is the mainstay of therapy. Bran in a dose of 10–25 grams/day can help relieve symptoms. It works in two ways: (a) to increase intraluminal bulk of undigested material and water; and (b) to produce a mild osmotic diarrhea through the breakdown of bran to short-chain fatty acids such as propionate and butyrate. The old teaching that recommends avoiding seeds and nuts that could lodge within a diverticulum no longer holds true.

3. Medication.

a. Bulk agents, such as psyllium hydrophilic mucilloid, work similarly to bran.

b. Antispasmodics, such as dicyclomine or propantheline,

are used for their anticholinergic effects. Their clinical efficacy, however, has not been proven in controlled trials.

IV. **Diverticular Bleeding**

A. Pathogenesis
1. Bleeding emanates from a single, noninflamed diverticulum. Since diverticula are in contact with the perforating vessels (vasa recta), local pressure can produce asymmetric thinning of a vessel's wall. The vessel may then rupture into the diverticulum, leading to hematochezia.
2. Bleeding occurs in 10% of patients with colonic diverticula. Most patients bleed only once; only 20–25% bleed a second time. With recurrent bleeding, however, the risk of a third bleed increases to 50%.
3. In 70% of cases of diverticular bleeding, the site of bleeding is a diverticulum in the right colon.

B. Clinical Features
Patients present with massive, painless hematochezia.

C. Differential Diagnosis
1. Arteriovenous malformations (AVMs).
2. Colon cancer.
3. Ischemic colitis.

D. Management
1. As with any bleeding patient, initial management is resuscitation and hemodynamic stabilization.
2. With massive hematochezia, it is necessary to rule out an upper gastrointestinal (UGI) source of hemorrhage by passage of a nasogastric tube.
3. Rigid sigmoidoscopy and anoscopy can rule out local sources of bleeding, such as hemorrhoids, and some extensive sources, such as infectious colitis or ulcerative colitis, and these examinations can also assess the severity of bleeding.
4. Since bleeding will stop spontaneously in 80% of cases, most patients can be observed without urgent diagnostic or invasive therapeutic maneuvers.
5. For the patient who continues to bleed, requiring transfusion, several diagnostic options are available, including radionuclide scanning, angiography, and endoscopy. (See Chapter 3.)

      6. There are also several therapeutic options in the patient with persistent diverticular bleeding. The choices include selective intraarterial infusion of vasopressin, angiographic embolization, or surgical resection.

V. Diverticulitis

  A. Pathogenesis

      1. Feces lodged in a diverticulum press on the diverticulum's mucosa, causing decreased blood flow and pressure necrosis of the mucosa. Microperforation ensues, with bacterial invasion of the pericolic tissues and development of a small intramural abscess, a pericolic abscess, or even peritonitis.

      2. Diverticulitis usually occurs in the sigmoid colon, where stool is more solid.

      3. Some authors report that up to 10–20% of patients with diverticula develop at least one episode of diverticulitis.

  B. Clinical and Laboratory Features

      1. Patients can present in three fashions:

        a. Acute. The typical triad of pain, fever, and left lower quadrant mass is the most common presentation. The abdominal pain is severe, radiates to the back, and is worse with bowel movements. Fever is almost always present. Patients may complain of dysuria and urgency, indicating bladder irritation from the inflamed sigmoid.

        b. Subacute. Self-limited disease, which spontaneously resolves with no therapy, or minimal therapy.

        c. Chronic. Sequelae of recurrent bouts of diverticulitis include obstructing stricture or fistulae.

      2. Hematochezia is distinctly uncommon in diverticulitis and is more suggestive of other diagnoses, especially perforating sigmoid cancer. Similarly, diarrhea is not a major symptom and should raise the possibility of colitis.

      3. Acutely ill patients will be tender in the left lower quadrant. Localized peritoneal signs and a tender palpable mass are usually present. Rectal exam may also reveal a tender mass anteriorly.

      4. Although gross bleeding is rare, stool testing will be positive for occult blood in 25% of cases.

      5. It is common to find leukocytosis with left shift. Abdominal x-ray can show obstruction or ileus. Urinalysis can confirm

suspected bladder irritation with the presence of microscopic hematuria.
C. Differential Diagnosis
   1. Perforating Colon Cancer. This can be a difficult differential diagnosis. Barium enema can reveal an intraluminal filling defect that is suggestive of cancer but is really an intramural abscess.
   2. Colitis.
D. Complications
   1. Free perforation and peritonitis.
   2. Abscess.
   3. Fistulae. Colovesical fistulae are the most common, especially in men, who have no uterus to act as a barrier to protect the bladder. Patients with this type of fistula are symptomatic with pneumaturia, fecaluria, and persistent or recurrent urinary infection. Coloenteric fistulae, by contrast, are usually asymptomatic.
   4. Obstruction. This complication occurs either acutely, secondary to edema and inflammation, or else late, secondary to fibrosis and stricture formation.
E. Management
   1. Initial management should be to stabilize the patient with intravenous fluids, bedrest, antibiotics, and nothing by mouth. Seventy to eighty-five percent of patients acutely ill with diverticulitis do well with medical management alone.
   2. The acutely ill patient generally should not be examined with a colonoscope or barium enema, since there is a risk of converting the initial microperforation into free perforation. Rigid sigmoidoscopic inspection using little or no air insufflation can be used to rule out active colitis. After 3–7 days of medical therapy, confirmation of the presumed diagnosis should be obtained with a barium enema.
   3. Patients with mild disease (classified on the basis of examination and laboratory values) may be treated as outpatients with oral antibiotics, either ampicillin or a second-generation cephalosporin. Severely ill patients should be treated in hospital with broad-spectrum intravenous antibiotics. The older treatment with ampicillin or a second-generation cephalosporin combined with an aminoglycoside and the anaerobic coverage of clindamycin or metronidazole has

largely been replaced by single agents such as Unisyn or cefoxitin. All patients should be treated for 7–10 days.

4. Urgent surgery is performed for free perforation, persistent abscess, or colonic obstruction. This surgery is usually performed in two stages. The first stage includes resection of the involved area, an end colostomy of the proximal colon, and oversewing the rectal stump (Hartmann's pouch). The second stage, performed after the patient makes a full recovery (4–6 weeks), takes down the colostomy and connects the colon to the rectal stump. Elective surgery, performed in one stage during an asymptomatic interval, is indicated for recurrent attacks of diverticulitis or chronic obstructive manifestations. The older three-stage procedure that began with simple diverting colostomy without resection is often ineffective and is not often recommended.

SUGGESTED READINGS

Almy TP, Howell DA: Diverticular diseases of the colon. *N Engl J Med* 302:324, 1980.

Painter NS, Burkitt DP: Diverticular disease of the colon, a 20th century problem. *Clin Gastroenterol* 4:3, 1975.

Chapter 16

Functional Disorders of Bowel Motility

Robert Shlien, M.D.
Blair S. Lewis, M.D.

I. Introduction

Motility of the gut is intrinsic to its proper function from mouth to anus. The intake of nutrients, their processing, and elimination of waste products all require movement. There are several diseases that are caused primarily by problems in motility. These include esophageal disorders, gastroparesis, intestinal pseudoobstruction, and constipation. We have included the irritable bowel syndrome among these, although the true etiology of this entity remains unknown. Disorders of esophageal motility are discussed in Chapter 2.

II. Gastroparesis

A. Pathophysiology
    1. Gastroparesis is nonobstructive delay in gastric emptying.
    2. Normally, the stomach has two separate regions performing the functions of storage, mixing, and emptying.
        a. The gastric fundus is one region. It has slow, nonperistaltic contractions useful for storage of solids and control of emptying of liquids.
        b. The gastric body and antrum grind food and then empty

it into the duodenum. The peristaltic contractions are controlled by a pacemaker located in the midbody of the stomach, which sets a minimum rate of three contractions per minute. This rate increases in response to feeding.

3. Function is also controlled by vagal and sympathetic nerves. Vagal fibers stimulate contractions and emptying.

B. Approach to the Patient

1. The predominant symptom is vomiting. Emesis can include undigested food and usually occurs hours after the meal.

   a. Other symptoms include new-onset brittleness in a patient with long-standing diabetes. With erratic absorption of nutrients due to abnormal gastric emptying, insulin coverage is often difficult to adjust.

2. Weight loss is common.

3. On examination, epigastric fullness can be felt. A succussion splash is indicative of retained liquids. Scars of previous abdominal surgery can give a clue as to possible previous vagotomy or gastric surgery.

4. Abdominal x-rays show an enlarged stomach. Metal clips near the spine may indicate a previous truncal vagotomy.

5. The primary role of diagnostic workup is to rule out the presence of outlet obstruction in these patients. The following special studies are of use:

   a. Upper Gastrointestinal (GI) Series. Although this can help in diagnosis by showing a dilated stomach with retained food and decreased or absent peristalsis, barium can remain in the stomach for a prolonged period, making further evaluation difficult. Emptying of liquid barium may be normal in spite of abnormal emptying of solids.

   b. Endoscopy. An excellent means of ruling out an anatomic obstruction from ulcer disease or neoplasm. Retained food after an 8–10 hour fast is indicative of abnormality.

   c. Barium Burger. A measure of gastric handling of solids.

   d. Gastric Emptying Scan. A radionuclide-labeled meal is given, usually eggs. The exact rate of emptying can be calculated.

C. Specific Causes
   1. Acute retention can occur following viral gastroenteritis and can be seen in diabetic ketoacidosis and sepsis as well as during use of total parenteral nutrition (TPN).
   2. Certain medications can also delay gastric emptying, for example, narcotics and tricyclic antidepressants.
   3. Diabetes is the most common cause of nonobstructive delay in gastric emptying.
      a. Thought to be secondary to vagal neuropathy.
      b. Associated with autonomic neuropathy symptoms.
      c. Difficult control of glycemia ensues.
      d. Abnormal fundal and antral motor function.
      e. Small intestine motor function preserved.
   4. Vagotomy following gastric surgery may cause stasis.
      a. May occur acutely postoperatively or may be chronic.
      b. Associated with both truncal and superselective vagotomy.
   5. A variety of other causes have been identified, including anorexia nervosa, gastric ulcer, muscular dystrophy, and dermatomyositis, to name a few.
   6. Idiopathic dysrhythmias are a new class of disorders, and not much is known about them at present.
      a. These are rare disorders. In one of them, termed *antral tachygastria*, a rapid pacemaker in the antrum prevents peristalsis.
      b. These disorders are associated with abnormal small bowel and colonic motility.
D. Therapy
   1. Metoclopramide, a dopaminergic drug with cholinergic effects, enhances peristalsis and lowers pyloric sphincter pressure. It also has antiemetic properties within the central nervous system. In the severely symptomatic patient, this medication can be given intravenously to assure absorption. Once gastric emptying is improved, the oral form can be administered.
   2. Bethanechol, a direct cholinergic agent. Though effective, it has common side effects of abdominal cramps and diarrhea.
   3. Surgery, whether pyloroplasty or gastroenterostomy, is usually of little value in patients with diabetes or with one

of the idiopathic dysrhythmias. Postvagotomy patients may be helped by one of these procedures.

4. Newer medications are presently under study.
   a. Domperidone acts similarly to metoclopramide but does not cross the blood-brain barrier; thus, extrapyramidal side effects are minimized.
   b. Cisapride is a potent stimulator not only of gastric emptying but also of small bowel and colonic motility.

III. Chronic Intestinal Pseudoobstruction

A. Definition

A syndrome characterized by signs and symptoms of bowel obstruction in the absence of a mechanical obstructing lesion. This is a chronic disorder. The acute form of ileus, or paralytic ileus, will not be discussed.

B. Classification

1. Probably a heterogeneous group of disorders.
   a. Different histologic appearance.
   b. The extent of involvement of the gastrointestinal tract varies.
   c. In some cases, there is involvement of other organs, such as the bladder.
   d. There seem to be both familial and sporadic forms.
2. The major differential classification is between primary idiopathic pseudoobstruction, and those cases that are secondary to diseases affecting the intestinal musculature or innervation.

C. Pathology

There are three major subtypes, based on pathologic features:

1. Neuropathic. Degeneration and swelling of the myenteric nerve plexus are seen.
2. Myopathic. Degeneration and vacuolization of muscle fibers are seen.
3. No histopathologic changes are noted in the third subtype.

D. Clinical Manifestations

1. The disease may affect the entire GI tract or just isolated segments.
2. The small bowel is most commonly affected.
3. Symptoms may be indistinguishable from those of mechanical organic obstruction.

4. Symptoms often begin in childhood or adolescence.
5. Patients usually have recurring episodes, and may have minor symptoms, or none at all, between episodes.
6. There is often marked abdominal distention, associated with pain and a change in bowel habits.
7. Pain may be very severe and is sometimes relieved by the passage of stool or gas, or by vomiting.
8. Weight loss of a significant degree is common.
9. Diarrhea may occur secondary to stasis of small bowel contents and bacterial overgrowth.
10. In the idiopathic form of the disease, familial involvement may be present in as many as one-third of patients.
11. Isolated colonic involvement may also occur. With this form of the disease, the patients have recurrent fecal impactions and constipation associated with delayed transit. Plain abdominal films often reveal a dilated colon.

E. Diagnosis
1. Mechanical obstruction must first be ruled out. The most common causes include adhesions, hernias, tumors, and intussusception.
2. In mechanical obstruction, obstipation is usually seen. Diarrhea is seen more frequently in pseudoobstruction.
3. Pseudoobstruction is also suggested when there is evidence of bladder or esophageal abnormalities, if onset is early in life, or if there is a positive family history.
4. The diagnosis can usually be made on the basis of radiologic studies and esophageal manometry. Manometry is abnormal in more than 80% of cases.
5. Once the diagnosis has been made, a search for systemic diseases causing the syndrome should be undertaken (Table 16.1). Secondary pseudoobstruction is more common than the idiopathic form.
   a. A careful history should be taken, looking for features that suggest collagen-vascular or endocrine disorders.
   b. A careful drug history should be taken.
   c. Physical exam should focus on features suggestive of the CREST syndrome (calcinosis, Raynaud's phenomenon, sclerodactyly, telangiectasia).
   d. Laboratory tests should include antinuclear antibody (ANA), rheumatoid factor, creatinine phosphokinase

Table 16.1.
Causes of Chronic Intestinal Pseudoobstruction

  I. Collagen vascular disease: progressive systemic sclerosis, dermatomyositis, systemic lupus erythematosus, polyarteritis nodosa.
 II. Amyloidosis.
III. Primary muscle diseases: muscular dystrophy, myotonic dystrophy.
 IV. Neurologic diseases: multiple sclerosis, Parkinson's disease, Hirschsprung's disease, spinal cord injury, Chagas's disease.
  V. Endocrine disorders: hypothyroidism, hyperthyroidism, hypoparathyroidism, diabetes mellitus, pheochromocytoma.
 VI. Drugs: opiates, antiparkinsonian drugs, phenothiazaines, clonidine, ganglion blockers, tricyclic antidepressants.
VII. Miscellaneous: porphyria, neoplasm with celiac plexus invasion, alcoholism, radiation enteritis.

        (CPK) (for muscular dystrophies), thyroid function tests, and fasting glucose.
  F. Treatment
      1. Treatment of chronic intestinal pseudoobstruction has been unsuccessful for the most part. Metoclopramide and cholinergic agents have been found to be ineffective.
      2. If there is suspicion of bacterial overgrowth, a 10–14 day trial of tetracycline can be given and may reduce some of the symptoms.
      3. Dietary manipulations, such as initiation of a diet low in fat, fiber, and lactose, has been recommended but is probably beneficial only in a small minority of these patients.
      4. Surgery should be avoided except as a last resort. It is helpful only in patients with segmental involvement.

IV. Constipation

  A. Pathophysiology
      1. Constipation is defined as hardness or infrequency of bowel movements.
      2. Causes.
          a. Mechanical Obstruction. When evaluating a patient with constipation, one is always concerned that it may be due to a mechanical obstruction such as a colonic cancer, polyp, or stricture.
          b. Diet. Low-fiber diet decreases colonic transit time and,

along with poor fluid intake, decreases the amount of water in stool, making it hard.

   c. Abnormal colonic motility can lead to constipation in two ways:

     i. Delayed transit time. This usually is secondary to metabolic causes such as:

       a. Medications. Analgesics, sedatives, oral iron, and antidepressants, among others.

       b. Diseases. Diabetes, hypothyroidism, hypercalcemia, Parkinson's disease.

       c. Pregnancy.

     ii. Prolonged storage of feces in the sigmoid colon.

       a. Irritable bowel disease.

       b. Diverticular disease.

       c. Neurologic causes, including lack of bowel training in the patient with multiple cerebrovascular accidents (CVAs) or mental retardation; and travel, stress, or depression.

   d. Anorectal Disorders. Anal fissures, perirectal abscess, and thrombosed external hemorrhoids all can lead to painful defecation and thus to avoidance of bowel movements.

   e. Neurologic Disorders. There are many neurologic causes, including spinal cord lesions, von Recklinghausen's disease, and Hirschsprung's disease.

     i. Hirschsprung's disease.

       a. Absence of neurons and resultant spasticity in the distal bowel.

       b. Constipation from birth.

       c. No stool on rectal exam.

       d. Barium enema shows dilated proximal colon.

       e. Diagnosis made by rectal biopsy and absence of neurons. Rectal manometry can also be diagnostic, with absence of relaxation of internal sphincter.

B. Approach to the Patient

   1. Before prescribing laxatives, the physician should evaluate each patient. A complete history and physical exam can help identify the cause of constipation. It is important to

know if this is an acute problem related to some medication, recent stress, or travel. If this is a chronic problem, a search for metabolic derangements may be in order. The rectal examination will assess anorectal disease and occult blood. Blood tests to determine thyroid function should be performed.

2. Extent of further evaluation is somewhat dictated by the age of the patient.

   a. In the pediatric population, Hirschsprung's disease must be considered, and a barium enema and rectal manometry or biopsy may be indicated.

   b. In the young adult, psychogenic causes are common. Still, a thorough history and physical exam should be done, and serum thyroid and calcium levels should be checked.

   c. In the older patient, it is important to exclude obstructive disease such as cancer or diverticular disease as a possible cause.

3. It should be remembered that symptoms may include not only less frequent bowel movements but also abdominal pain and nausea. Fecal impaction can lead to overflow diarrhea or stercoral ulceration and rectal bleeding. Rectal prolapse, hemorrhoids, ischemic colitis, and sigmoid volvulus all may result from severe constipation.

C. Therapy

1. If an underlying cause can be elicited, it should be treated, perhaps as simply as by stopping certain medications.

2. A diet high in fiber should be advised, as well as the intake of plenty of fluids and the addition of daily exercise.

3. Laxatives work in different ways and are useful for the short term, but long-term dependence should be discouraged. Types of laxatives are:

   a. Stool Softeners. These medications (e.g., Colace, Surfak) are surfactants. They allow water uptake by fatty material in stool, making the stool softer. These medications are good for mild, acute constipation and also are recommended for use in patients who should not strain with bowel movements, such as the post-myocardial infarction patient or the patient after rectal surgery.

b. Bulk Agents. These medications (e.g., Metamucil, Hydrocil, Effersyllium) are water-soluble polysaccharides that absorb water and increase in size. Bulk agents are ideal for the treatment of chronic constipation.

c. Osmotic agents or saline laxatives are nonabsorbable salts that are hyperosmotic. They are very effective cathartics in the patient with acute constipation or the patient who is about to undergo a colonic examination. These agents, however, do entail a risk of dehydration.
   i. Magnesium salts.
      a. Hydroxide (milk of magnesia).
      b. Sulfate (epsom salt).
      c. Citrate (citrate of magnesia).
   ii. Sodium phosphate.

d. Irritants or stimulants are medications that stimulate colonic motility and secretion of water and sodium. Patients may develop abdominal cramps with their use.
   i. Anthraquinone derivatives include cascara and senna. Extended use of these natural agents can lead to melanosis coli.
   ii. Phenolphthalein is also an irritant (Ex-Lax, Evac-U-Gen, Correctol).
   iii. Bisacodyl (Dulcolax) is another irritant agent.
   iv. Castor oil is metabolized to ricinoleic acid, which then exerts its irritant effect.

e. Lubricants such as mineral oil are excellent therapy for fecal impaction. They can be administered orally or as retention enemas. The oil is adsorbed by the stool, making it soft. Oral administration may be complicated by aspiration and lipoid pneumonia in the elderly or infirm patient, especially at bedtime or when lying down.

f. Other agents include:
   i. Lactulose, a nonabsorbable disaccharide leading to an osmotic diarrhea much like that caused by milk ingestion in the lactase-deficient patient. Though used more routinely for hepatic encephalopathy, this medication may also be used in the treatment of constipation.
   ii. Glycerin suppository, a mild irritant when placed in the rectum. It is also hyperosmolar, and these two properties cause a bowel movement to occur.

V. Irritable Bowel Syndrome (IBS)

A. Definition

A syndrome of abdominal pain accompanied by altered bowel habits and unexplained by organic pathology.

B. Pathophysiology

1. The etiology is unknown. However, it is suspected that IBS is a motility disorder. Since IBS is a syndrome and not a specific disease, there are most likely many subgroups of patients.

2. Experimental findings suggestive of disordered motility in IBS patients include the following:

   a. Lower threshold to pain with balloon distention of the rectum.

   b. Increased slow wave (3 cycle/minute) electrical activity.

   c. Increased motor response of the colon to stimulatory drugs (cholecystokinin (CCK), cholinergics) and food.

   d. Increased frequency of high-amplitude pressure waves in the colon of patients with pain-predominant IBS.

3. Psychosocial factors are clearly important.

   a. Symptoms are usually exacerbated by stress.

   b. Multiple studies have shown an association with various personality factors, and an increase in the incidence of chronic anxiety, depression, and hysteria in patients with IBS. These personality factors, however, may be determinants of which patients persist in seeking medical help for their complaints, rather than integral features of IBS itself. The symptoms of IBS may, in fact, be prevalent in nearly 15% of the "normal" population.

C. Clinical Features

1. Abdominal pain associated with diarrhea, constipation, or alternating diarrhea and constipation.

   a. Pain is usually poorly localized but is more often noted in the lower abdomen.

   b. Pain is described as aching or cramping, and is often relieved by passage of flatus or stool.

2. Diarrhea may be described as increased frequency of stools or decreased consistency (loose or semiformed). However, objective increase in fecal volume is rarely present. Increased frequency of stools is often noted after meals, during stress, and upon arising in the morning.

3. Constipation may be described as a decrease in the frequency of bowel movements, passage of hard scybalous (pebble-like) stools, or a sensation of incomplete evacuation of the rectum. Patients may also note passage of thin, soft, pencil-like stools.
4. Increased passage of mucus per rectum with either flatus or stool may also be noted.
5. Upper GI complaints include nausea, vomiting, dyspepsia, increased gas, and frequent belching.
6. Other symptoms may include fatigue, headache, depression, and multiple somatic complaints.

D. Diagnosis
1. History.
   a. Symptoms that are reported more commonly in IBS patients and suggest the diagnosis include the following:
      i. Looser or more frequent bowel movements with the onset of pain.
      ii. Relief of pain with a bowel movement.
      iii. Abdominal distention.
      iv. The presence of increased mucus or a sensation of incomplete evacuation of the rectum.
   b. Symptoms or signs that are *not* characteristic of IBS and should lead to investigation for other pathology are:
      i. Recent onset of symptoms, especially in an elderly patient.
      ii. Pain that is not associated with a change in bowel habits.
      iii. Fever.
      iv. Gross or occult blood in the stool.
      v. Nocturnal awakening with symptoms of pain or diarrhea.
      vi. Weight loss.
      vii. Greasy or fatty stools.
      viii. Abnormal blood studies.
   c. Questions about psychosocial factors and sources of stress are important.
   d. A history of increased symptoms associated with lactose intake should be sought. Lactose intolerance may be confused with IBS or may exist concurrently with it. A

lactose tolerance test or at least a trial of a lactose-free diet may be helpful in certain cases.

e. Other dietary factors may also be important, such as excessive use of alcohol, coffee, or diet items that contain sorbitol.

f. Patients should also be questioned about laxative use. Laxative abusers may complain of diarrhea, yet deny use. In addition, some patients complaining of constipation will have a long history of laxative use and a hypomotile "cathartic colon."

g. It is important to question the patient about his or her reason for seeking help at the time of consultation. Studies have shown that as many as 15% of the general population have the symptoms of IBS, but less than half of these seek a physician. Death of a relative or fear of cancer rather than severity of symptoms may be the reason the patient has decided to see a physician.

2. Physical exam is usually normal in IBS patients. Occasionally tenderness may be present, especially over the sigmoid colon. Patients may also complain of increased pain during the rectal examination.

3. Diagnostic Studies.

a. Initial screening.

    i. Complete history and physical exam.

    ii. Pelvic examination.

    iii. Examination of stool for ova and parasites, and culture for bacterial pathogens.

    iv. Complete blood cell count (CBC), urinalysis, erythrocyte sedimentation rate (ESR), routine blood chemistries.

    v. Flexible or rigid sigmoidoscopy.

b. Further diagnostic studies should be individualized for each patient and determined by the following:

    i. Any positive findings on the initial study.

    ii. Predominant symptoms (pain, constipation, or diarrhea).

    iii. The age of the patient and chronicity of the complaints.

    iv. The severity of the patient's symptoms.

    c. As a general guideline, the following tests should be considered under the circumstances below:

      i. Patients over age 40 with recent onset of symptoms: barium enema.

      ii. Patients with symptoms that are persistent or worsening: barium enema and upper GI series with small bowel follow-through.

      iii. Patients predominantly with abdominal pain: abdominal ultrasound or computed tomography (CT) scan.

      iv. Worsening or persistent diarrhea: barium enema, upper GI and small bowel, malabsorption work-up, thyroid function tests. Also consider gastrin, 5-hydroxyindoleacetic acid (5HIAA), vasoactive intestinal polypeptide (VIP) tests.

4. Differential Diagnosis.

    a. Infectious Disorders.

      i. Parasitic—*Giardia lamblia, Entamoeba histolytica.*

      ii. Bacterial—*Salmonella, Campylobacter, Yersinia, Clostridium difficile.*

    b. Inflammatory bowel disease.

    c. Diverticular disease of the colon.

    d. Drug use.

      i. Cathartics.

      ii. Antacids containing magnesium.

      iii. Other drugs (quinidine, etc.).

    e. Malabsorption/maldigestion.

      i. Celiac sprue.

      ii. Pancreatic insufficiency.

    f. Psychiatric disorders.

      i. Depression.

      ii. Somatization.

    g. Neoplastic disorders.

      i. Adenocarcinoma of the colon.

      ii. Villous adenoma.

      iii. Endocrine tumors: gastrinoma, VIPoma, carcinoid.

    h. Metabolic disorders.

      i. Hypothyroidism (constipation) and hyperthyroidism (diarrhea).

      ii. Diabetes mellitus.

      iii. Lactase deficiency.

E. Therapy
  1. Goals of Therapy.
     a. Patient's understanding of the condition.
        i. It is important to stress that there is no evidence to suggest a more serious disorder (i.e., cancer). Then the patient should be made to understand that IBS is a real disorder. It is often helpful to explain that the bowel is sensitive to stimuli such as stress, hormones, and possibly dietary factors.
        ii. Although psychological factors are important, the patient should not be told that this is an emotional or psychiatric disorder. Psychiatric referral is indicated only in certain specific instances.
     b. Adaptation of the patient to the condition and modification of those factors that exacerbate symptoms.
        i. The patient should understand that "cure" is not a realistic expectation but that the goal of treatment will be to try to ameliorate symptoms to the point of tolerability.
        ii. Identification of stress factors in the patient's life may clarify the relationship of stressful events to exacerbation of symptoms. This is often helpful to the patient in coping when symptoms are worse, and may initiate some modifications in life-style to reduce stress.
     c. Amelioration of predominant symptoms (pain, diarrhea, or constipation).
  2. Diet.
     a. Diet is the most common form of therapy used in IBS. Increased fiber, in the form of either bran, or a commercial preparation such as psyllium or methylcellulose, is probably effective. Although some controlled studies have not shown benefit, side effects are minimal.
     b. Fiber shortens intestinal transit time, thus probably benefiting patients with constipation. It may also help patients with diarrhea by adding bulk and consistency to the stool.
     c. Bran can be started at a dose of 1 tablespoon t.i.d. and gradually increased to a total of 16 grams/day (2 tablespoons t.i.d.). Initially patients may complain of bloating or diarrhea, so it is essential to warn them of this problem

in advance; but they should be encouraged to continue the diet therapy for at least 3 weeks before concluding that it is not effective. Bran or psyllium wafers, which are somewhat more palatable than powdered forms, are also available, as well as the many commercial fiber preparations (Metamucil, Konsyl, etc.).

   d. Foods that are high in undigestible carbohydrate, such as beans, cabbage, and brussels sprouts, should be avoided.

   e. Patients with suspected lactase deficiency should have a trial of a lactose-free diet.

   f. Elimination diets have some proponents. However, there are still not enough data to support their general use.

3. Drugs.

   a. There are few well-designed double blind studies that assess the efficacy of drug therapy in IBS. Since these patients are high placebo-responders, one must be very cautious in drawing conclusions from uncontrolled studies.

   b. Anticholinergics may be used in patients with predominant constipation or pain. Dosage is limited by side effects of dry mouth and blurred vision, especially in elderly patients. Usually these drugs are given before meals and at bedtime. No particular drug in this category has been shown to be most efficacious.

     i. Dicyclomine can be started at a dose of 10 mg q.i.d. and increased to 20 mg q.i.d. (about half this dose in elderly patients).

     ii. Alternatively, propantheline can be given, 15 mg 30 minutes before meals and 30 mg at bedtime.

   c. Antidiarrheals.

     i. Mild diarrhea may respond to bulking agents (hydrophilic colloids such as psyllium or methylcellulose).

     ii. More severe diarrhea may require diphenoxylate (Lomotil) 1 or 2 tabs (2.5 or 5 mg) every 4–6 hours, or loperamide (Imodium) 1 or 2 tabs (2 or 4 mg) every 8 hours.

   d. Antidepressants. Are especially helpful in patients who show clinical signs of depression such as weight loss, sleep disturbance, or family history of depression. Usually given in a single nighttime dose, e.g., amitryiptyline (Elavil) 25–50 mg.

e. Analgesics.
   i. Opiates should not be used to treat pain, as they worsen constipation and are potentially addictive.
   ii. Acute exacerbations of pain may respond to anticholinergics. In addition, a heating pad or warm baths may partially alleviate pain during these acute episodes.
   iii. Nonsteroidal antiinflammatory agents can be tried for chronic pain.
f. Antiflatulents. None has been shown to be effective. Simethicone (2–4 tabs) or activated charcoal tabs have been tried.
g. Antianxiety Agents. Long-term use of benzodiazepines should be avoided, and management of stress should focus on nondrug therapy.

4. Other Therapy.
   a. Psychiatric referral should be infrequent but may be necessary in certain instances:
      i. If there are signs of marked depression or other psychiatric disorders.
      ii. If the patient is unable to function because of the symptoms.
      iii. If the physician and patient agree that psychotherapy may help the patient cope with stress. The patient should understand that referral to a psychiatrist does not represent rejection by the primary physician, nor a failure to take his or her symptoms seriously.
   b. Biofeedback, hypnosis, exercise, and relaxation techniques have all been tried, with ancedotal reports of success. If facilities are available, one of these techniques may be used, but it is important that the physician maintain overall control of the patient's care.

SUGGESTED READINGS

Harvey RF, Salih SY, Read AE: Organic and functional disorders in 2,000 gastroenterology outpatients. *Lancet* 1:632–634, 1983.

Whitehead WE, Schuster MM: The irritable bowel, stress, and the colon. In Kirsner JB, Shorter RG (eds): *Diseases of the Colon, Rectum, and Anal Canal.* Baltimore, Williams & Wilkins, 1988, chap 21.

Chapter 17

Common Anorectal Disorders

Nathaniel Cohen, M.D.

I. Introduction

Anorectal complaints tend to be a source of embarrassment to most patients. In addition, patients frequently are afraid of what the physician may find or may do to them. Many physicians also dislike discussing these complaints and performing the rectal examination and sigmoidoscopy necessary to accurately diagnose and treat the condition. It is essential for the physician to overcome these aversions, take a detailed history, and do a careful examination.

II. History

A. Pain

The type and timing of the pain frequently give a clue as to the diagnosis. Anal fissure pain usually has its onset at defecation and usually subsides gradually over minutes to hours. An abscess of the rectum usually is associated with a steadily increasing, constant pain until the abscess drains. Hemorrhoids usually produce intermittent rectal or perianal discomfort, but severe pain occurs only with thrombosis. Proctitis can be produced by infectious, ischemic, and idiopathic causes and has anal discomfort as one of its symptoms; as well as tenesmus.

Proctalgia fugax usually presents as severe rectal pain of short duration, which can awaken the patient from sleep.

B. Bleeding

Rectal bleeding is a very common complaint that must always be taken seriously and investigated. Characteristically, the bleeding is bright red. Although hemorrhoids are by far the most common cause of fresh red rectal bleeding, other causes such as tumors (benign or malignant), proctitis, foreign body trauma, fistulas, and rectal ulcers must always be ruled out. The mere presence of hemorrhoids does not preclude the possibility that one of these other conditions may be the cause of rectal bleeding.

C. Pruritus

Itching of the anus or perianal area is a common complaint. Although most patients attribute the symptom to hemorrhoids, it can be due to many causes, including overzealous cleaning, diarrhea, rectal discharge and moisture, moniliasis, pinworms, scabies, sensitivity to topical medications or perfumed toilet tissue, and systemic conditions such as diabetes, lymphoma, or liver disease.

D. Mass

Although hemorrhoids are the most common cause of rectal mass or protrusion, other causes, such as prolapsed polyps, prolapsed rectum, and rectal malignancies, must always be considered.

III. Physical Examination

A careful examination is mandatory in determining the cause of a patient's complaints or symptoms. The patient must be relaxed and reassured that there will be little if any pain involved. An ordinary examination table is adequate, and there should be good light. The left lateral decubitus position is usually utilized.

First, the perianal area should be thoroughly inspected, looking for any abnormalities such as skin tags, external hemorrhoids, anal fistula opening, fecal soiling, excoriations secondary to pruritus, skin changes, swelling of thrombosed hemorrhoids, or any sign of a malignancy. Next, the buttocks should be retracted to visualize the anal verge and part of the anal canal. Palpation of the area may show evidence of an abscess with tenderness or heat, or a fistulous tract may feel like a cord-like segment that extrudes pus from its external opening when pressure is applied.

Digital examination should then be performed with a well-lubricated glove or finger cot. Touching the anus causes the sphincter to contract, so a few moments must be allowed for it to relax before the finger is inserted, using gentle steady pressure. In addition to feeling for masses and tenderness, one should always note sphincter tone and make some assessment of the feel of the mucosa. The material adhering to the finger always should be inspected and then examined for occult blood.

IV. Endoscopic Examination

The introduction of the fiberoptic proctosigmoidoscope has meant a major advance in the care of patients, but it does have some limitations, and there is still a place for anoscopy and rigid proctosigmoidoscopy. If there is any doubt as to the findings in the anal area, the anoscope is the instrument to use. It permits excellent visualization and a larger lumen for instrumentation, suction, and cleaning the lumen. In addition, hemostasis with direct pressure by swabs is easily attained. The rigid proctosigmoidoscope has the same advantages and is 25 cm in length. However, the bowel must be made to conform to the straight scope. It frequently is not possible to advance beyond the sigmoid bend, with about 18 cm inserted.

The fiberoptic proctosigmoidoscope comes in lengths ranging from 30 to 60 cm, but the longer versions are becoming the instruments of choice. Most patients prefer it to the rigid proctosigmoidoscope because the examination is usually more comfortable. It is carried out on an ordinary examining table with the patient lying in the left lateral decubitus position. All the necessary ancillary equipment should be readily available for biopsy, culture, polypectomy, and hemostasis. (See Chapter 21.)

V. Common Anorectal Disorders

A. Hemorrhoids

Although hemorrhoids formerly were thought by many to be simple varicose veins of the rectum, it now is thought that they are normally present in everyone and are separate bulky cushions of specialized submucosal connective tissue that help effect complete closure of the anus. Those present above the dentate line are called internal hemorrhoids, and those below are called external hemorrhoids. They are important only if they produce symptoms. Enlargement, displacement downward, thrombosis, or trauma can produce symptoms such as bleeding, pain, or protrusion. Although internal hemorrhoids are the most common cause of bright red rectal bleeding, pathology higher in the colon must be excluded, especially in older patients, even though they may have obvious, symptomatic bleeding hemorrhoids. Constipation, diarrhea, and straining at stools are the usual factors involved in hemorrhoids becoming symptomatic. Thrombosed external hemorrhoids, when they resolve, develop into perianal skin tags, which become irritated by poor anal hygiene and perspiration.

Most cases of hemorrhoids can be treated medically with good results. Sitz baths, good anal hygiene, and avoidance of extremes of bowel activity are the basics of medical management. There is no proven role for topical corticosteroids, but some authorities advocate use of 1% hydrocortisone cream to promote lubrication and anti-inflammatory activity and to stop anal itching. A high fiber intake plus a lot of liquids will help with bowel movements and decrease the bleeding and prolapse that often occur. Invasive modalities such as injection sclerotherapy, rubber band ligation, infrared coagulation, cryosurgery, and laser coagulation all have their adherents. Operative hemorrhoidectomy is still necessary in patients who are either unsuitable or fail to respond to these treatments.

B. Fissures

Anal fissures are the commonest cause of anal pain. They are short (frequently less than 1 cm long) tears or ulcers of the anoderm between the anal opening and the dentate line. They are thought to result from trauma to the distal anal canal, for example by passage of bulky, large, hard stools. Their locations are characteristic, with 95–99% of men and 80–90% of women having them in the posterior midline. Almost all the rest are in the anterior midline. If a fissure is not in either the posterior or anterior midline, then inflammatory bowel disease must be ruled out.

Typically, anal pain due to fissures is described as burning, stinging, or tearing occurring with defecation and gradually subsiding within an hour. It is frequently associated with a small amount of bright red blood on the toilet tissue. Fissures can often be visualized without instruments by lifting the buttocks apart and having the patient bear down. A gentle digital examination with pressure away from the fissure will reveal spasm or tension of the anus. When the fissure is chronic, one may find a hypertrophic anal papilla proximal to it or a sentinel skin tag distal to it. Acute fissures will usually heal if the diet is changed to ensure soft, formed stools. Care must be used in prescribing local anesthetic agents because patients often become sensitive or allergic to them. If the fissure becomes chronic, then surgery is usually indicated. The operation of choice is internal sphincterotomy, since this procedure will allow most fissures to heal without being excised. The surgery must be done by an experienced anorectal surgeon in order to preserve anal continence.

C. Fistulas and Abscesses

Another common cause of anal pain is an anorectal abscess, which frequently produces steady, throbbing pain and on examination is a tender, red perianal swelling. It is thought to result from an infection of an anal crypt. It may sometimes drain spontaneously, with prompt pain relief. One must always be sure to rule out more serious disease, such as inflammatory bowel disease or tumor, as the underlying cause. When the abscess ruptures, it may track and the resulting fistula may then become chronic. The external opening of the fistula can usually be seen, and a bead of pus can often be expressed from it. Incision and adequate drainage is the treatment of choice for an anorectal abscess, with the addition of appropriate antibiotics if there is superimposed extensive cellulitis. Despite drainage, 50% of treated patients go on to develop fistulas. The abscess should be drained as close to the anus as possible, so that if a fistula forms it will be short. Surgery is usually necessary to cure a fistula.

D. Rectal Prolapse

Rectal prolapse is the circumferential descent of the rectum through the anal sphincter. It occurs most frequently in children less than 2 years old and in the elderly, especially in women. In children, the prolapse usually involves just mucosa and therefore is only a partial prolapse. In the elderly, a complete prolapse also occurs, with the entire thickness of the rectal wall protruding through the anus. The partial prolapse in children is self-limiting and usually is treated by manually reducing the prolapse and maintaining the reduction by strapping the buttocks together. Treatment of partial prolapse in adults is similar to that of hemorrhoids, using ligation with rubber bands, cryodestruction of the redundant mucosa, or surgical excision of the prolapsed mucosa. Controversy exists as to the surgical procedure of choice for complete rectal prolapse, and the final decision should be left to the surgeon, depending on his or her experience.

E. Fecal Impaction

Fecal impaction is frequently caused by overuse of narcotics, prolonged bed rest, or postoperative constipation. As feces accumulate in the rectum, the mass may harden as fecal fluids are absorbed or excreted. The hard mass of feces then becomes so large that it cannot be passed. Sometimes it may present as paradoxical diarrhea and incontinence when liquid and soft stool pass around the hard fecal mass. This diagnosis should be entertained whenever a postoperative patient, especially if elderly, develops "diarrhea." The diagnosis is usually confirmed by simple digital rectal examination. The best therapy is prevention. Once impaction has developed, evacuation should be attained with a minimum of trauma. Oral laxatives and tap water enemas are usually sufficient. In more difficult cases, the next step is to try stool softeners and warm oil retention enemas. If these do not work, then digital disimpaction becomes necessary. Once the patient is disimpacted, preventive measures including diet and laxatives become mandatory in order to avoid recurrences.

SUGGESTED READING

Corman M (ed): *Colon and Rectal Surgery*, ed 2. Philadelphia, JB Lippincott, 1989.

Chapter 18

Cancer of the Gastrointestinal Tract

Blair S. Lewis, M.D.

I. Esophageal Cancer

A. Epidemiology
1. There is an increased risk of esophageal cancer in patients who are male, black, smokers, or alcoholics, or who have a history of lye ingestion or radiotherapy, as well as in those who have a Barrett's esophagus, Plummer-Vinson syndrome, or tylosis (a rare hereditary disease with diffuse keratosis of the palms and soles).
2. There is a high incidence in Asian countries.
3. Prognosis is poor, with 5-year survival only 3–6%.

B. Pathology
1. Ninety percent of primary esophageal cancers are squamous carcinomas. Although adenocarcinomas constitute another 5% of primary esophageal cancers, the vast majority of adenocarcinomas encountered in the esophagus are actually gastric adenocarcinomas of the fundus growing up into the esophagus.
2. Esophageal cancer metastasizes early, because the esophagus has no tunica serosa to contain the tumor. The cancer metastasizes to the lungs and liver as well as along the path of lymph drainage. The upper third of the esophagus drains to the cervical lymph nodes, the middle third to the tra-

cheobronchial nodes, and the lower third to the gastric and celiac nodes.

C. Signs and Symptoms
1. Most patients present with symptoms of progressive dysphagia, initially to solids and ultimately to liquids. The diagnosis must be strongly suspected in any patient older than 40 years presenting with new-onset dysphagia.
2. Patients may also have pain, either odynophagia or back pain. Back pain is usually indicative of tumor extension and unresectability.
3. With a partially obstructing esophageal lesion, patients also experience weight loss and recurrent aspiration. Recurrent pneumonia should also raise the possibility of a tracheoesophageal fistula due to the tumor.

D. Diagnosis
1. Barium swallow shows an asymmetric, irregular narrowing.
2. Esophagoscopy, either rigid or flexible, can provide the diagnosis by biopsy or cytology.
3. Computed tomography (CT) scan can help measure tumor spread and thereby help to determine if the cancer is resectable.
4. ^{67}Gallium, which is picked up by squamous tumors, is also used to determine cancer spread.

E. Therapy
1. Curative therapy is surgical, with or without concomitant radiotherapy. Surgical resection includes esophagectomy with gastric pull-up when feasible, or else colonic or small bowel interposition when necessary.
2. Many different palliative therapies are used. Partial tumor ablation by endoscopic laser or bipolar tumor probe allows the patient to continue eating. Esophageal stent placement is also possible and is most commonly utilized in cases of tracheoesophageal fistula. Surgery and radiotherapy can also be used for palliation.

II. <u>Gastric Cancer</u>

A. Epidemiology

1. Decreasing incidence in the United States since 1940. Greatest incidence in Japan.
2. Risk Factors.
   a. Chronic benign gastric ulcer is suspected but not proven to be a risk factor.
   b. Achlorhydria is thought to predispose to cancer after many years by allowing bacterial overgrowth to produce carcinogenic metabolites.
      i. Partial gastrectomy.
      ii. Atrophic gastritis.
      iii. Pernicious anemia.
   c. Acanthosis nigricans, hyperpigmentation and keratosis of skin folds occurring spontaneously, carries an increased risk of any gastrointestinal (GI) malignancy, with gastric cancer accounting for 40% of the associated cancers.
   d. Dermatomyositis is associated with GI malignancies, 18% of which are gastric cancers.
   e. Gastric polyps, both hyperplastic and adenomatous, carry increased risk for cancer in the noninvolved mucosa.
   f. Blood group A is a risk factor for gastric cancer.
3. Poor prognosis, with 5-year survival of 10%, except for "early" form (see below).

B. Pathology
Adenocarcinoma, characterized pathologically by the presence of signet ring cells, takes many different forms.
1. Early gastric cancer is a common entity in Japan, where gastric cancer is prevalent and mass screening is performed. This type of cancer is defined as being limited to the mucosa or submucosa and has a 95% 5-year survival. These cancers are classified into three types: I is protruded, II is superficial, and III is excavated. Type II is further divided into three subtypes: subtype IIa is elevated, IIb is flat, and IIc is depressed.
2. Advanced cancer is the most common type seen in the United States. The Borrman classification divides these cancers into four types: (a) polypoid lesions, usually located in the fundus; (b) ulcerated, noninfiltrating lesions; (c) ulcerated infiltrating lesions, usually in the antrum; and (d) dif-

fusely infiltrating lesions, including linitis plastica.

3. Linitis plastica, also called "leather bottle stomach," is a submucosal tumor spreading diffusely and associated with a large desmoplastic reaction. The stomach, particularly the antrum, becomes narrowed and nondistensible. These tumors have the worst prognosis.

4. Superficial spreading cancer is another variant in which the cancer spreads laterally within the mucosa and submucosa without deep invasion. These tumors have a 95% 5-year survival, although up to 18% of patients have lymph node involvement with tumor at the time of surgery.

C. Signs and Symptoms

1. The diagnosis should be suspected whenever an elderly patient presents with symptoms of ulcer disease or outlet obstruction. Gastric outlet obstruction is characterized by persistent nausea and vomiting and, classically, regurgitation of food more than 4 hours after ingestion.

2. Patients may present without symptoms referable to the stomach, but with weight loss, symptoms of anemia, or a positive test for fecal occult blood.

D. Diagnosis

1. Upper GI series reveals a gastric mass or ulcer. There are radiographic guidelines to help determine if an ulcer is malignant or benign. Malignancy is indicated when the ulcer is within the stomach wall, within a gastric mass, or has irregular borders. Many gastric ulcers are indeterminate by barium studies.

2. Upper endoscopy with biopsy and cytology is usually effective in determining if cancer exists in a gastric ulcer.

3. Abdominal CT scan is useful in determining tumor spread.

E. Therapy

1. Surgery is necessary for cure. Surgical resection can also be employed for palliation in the patient with gastric outlet obstruction or persistent bleeding.

2. Chemotherapy is used for palliation in incurable cases. Combination therapy shows the greatest response, especially when adriamycin is included as one of the agents. FAM (5-FU, adriamycin, and mitomycin C) shows the greatest promise, with response rates of 40–50%.

III. Small Bowel Cancers

A. Epidemiology
1. Cancer of the small bowel is uncommon, accounting for less than 5% of all GI tract malignancies.
2. The risk of developing cancer of the small intestine is increased by the presence of sprue, familial polyposis, dermatitis herpetiformis, immunodeficiency, or Crohn's disease (ileitis) of very long duration.
3. There are four major types of primary small bowel cancer.
   a. Carcinoid tumors account for 1.5% of all GI tract cancers (see below).
   b. Adenocarcinoma tends to occur proximally, with 90% of lesions in the duodenum or jejunum within 20 cm of the ligament of Treitz; adenocarcinoma of the ileum is rarely encountered except in cases of long-standing ileitis.
   c. Lymphoma tends to occur distally in the distal jejunum or ileum.
   d. Leiomyosarcoma can occur anywhere in the small bowel and is the most common bleeding malignant small bowel tumor.
B. Signs and Symptoms
1. Intermittent small bowel obstruction is the most common presentation.
2. Patients may present with abdominal pain, diarrhea, or weight loss, or an abdominal mass may be found incidentally on examination.
C. Diagnosis
1. Isolated lesions of the small intestine can be difficult to visualize on a small bowel series. Enteroclysis, introducing barium and air directly into the small intestine through a long tube, may visualize individual loops of intestine and thus aid in diagnosis.
2. Laparoscopy or exploratory surgery is sometimes required to make the diagnosis.
D. Therapy
1. Surgical resection is necessary, especially in patients with small bowel obstruction.
2. Treatment of lymphoma with radiation or chemotherapy

raises the risk of small bowel perforation due to tumor necrosis.

E. Carcinoid Tumors

1. Carcinoid tumors originate from chromaffin cells of Kulchitsky in the crypts of Lieberkühn. These are tumors of so-called APUD cells (amine-precursor uptake and decarboxylation).

2. Although these tumors can occur anywhere in the body including lung, pancreas, and biliary tract, 90% are found within the GI tract. The appendix is the most common site, followed by terminal ileum and rectum.

3. These tumors are slow-growing, often allowing more than 10-year survival, even in patients with known liver metastases. Frequency of metastases increases with increasing size of the primary tumor, reaching 50% for primary tumors between 1 and 2 cm and 80% for those >2 cm. Liver and mesentery are common sites for metastases. Liver metastases may produce carcinoid syndrome. Mesenteric metastases may become fibrotic and cicatrize, leading to shortening and fixation of the small bowel. Appendiceal tumors rarely metastasize.

4. Carcinoid syndrome refers to the systemic effects of active agents released by the tumor. These signs and symptoms include diarrhea, abdominal pain, flushing, cyanosis, bronchospasm, valvular heart disease (thickening of the tricuspid and pulmonic valves), and telangiectasias. These effects are mainly due to serotonin released by the tumor. Other agents made by the tumors include histamine, catecholamines, kinins, adrenocorticotropic hormone (ACTH), and melanocyte-stimulating hormone. The syndrome occurs only when these agents are released into the general circulation, either from liver metastases or else from primary extraintestinal sites like the lung. The syndrome does not occur with isolated small bowel tumors, since the released hormones pass into the portal circulation and are quickly degraded by the liver.

   a. Diagnosis is made by finding elevated levels of a serotonin metabolite, 5-hydroxyindoleacetic acid (5-HIAA), in a 24-hour urine collection. Certain medications and foods can alter normal serotonin levels and thus yield misleading results. Bananas, pineapples, and walnuts, for example, increase serotonin levels, while phenothiazines, such as Compazine and Thorazine, lower serotonin levels.

b. Once carcinoid syndrome is present, curative surgery is not possible and therapy is directed at controlling symptoms. Medical therapy with somatostatin or its analogue, Sandostatin (SMS 201-995), exerts its effect by inhibiting hormone secretion. Sandostatin controls flushing and disease. Serotonin antagonists, such as methysergide or cyproheptadine, can be effective in controlling disease and other abdominal complaints. It should be noted that methysergide (Sansert) has severe side effects associated with prolonged use. These effects include retroperitoneal fibrosis, hypotension, and fluid retention. Chemotherapy and embolization of hepatic metastases are also part of palliation. Surgery generally does not play a role in carcinoid tumors with metastases. Surgery cannot cure the tumor once metastases have occurred, and surgery is made more difficult due to the cicatrized mesentery. Furthermore, surgery and anesthesia raise the risk of precipitating a carcinoid crisis with massive and sometimes fatal release of vasoactive agents.

IV. Colon Cancer

A. Epidemiology
1. The most common GI malignancy and the second most common cancer in the United States. There are 130,000 new cases and 60,000 deaths annually.
2. A "disease of Western civilization," with a very low incidence in underdeveloped countries. Western diets high in fat and low in fiber are thought to play a role in this difference.
3. The risk for colon cancer increases with increasing age, beginning at age 45 on average and doubling every 10 years until it peaks at age 75. There is an equal distribution in men and women.
4. Two-thirds of cancers occur in the left colon. The overall

distribution is: rectum 22%, sigmoid 35%, descending colon 6%, transverse colon 13%, ascending colon 8%, and cecum 15%.

5. The risk of developing colon cancer is increased in patients with a family history of colon cancer or multiple polyposis, or with a personal past history of colon polyps or cancer, inflammatory bowel disease, or female genital cancer.

   a. History of colon cancer, even surgically cured, carries a fourfold increase in risk of a subsequent new colon cancer, representing a lifetime risk of 15%.

   b. History of female genital cancer (cancer of the breast, cervix, ovary) carries a three-fold increase in risk, or a 7–20% lifetime risk.

   c. Family history of colon cancer in first degree-relatives also triples the risk. These cancers tend to be more right-sided and to occur in younger patients.

   d. Patients with ulcerative colitis have a risk for colon cancer beginning after 8–10 years of colitis, and this risk runs about 0.5% per year thereafter, approaching 10% by the 30th year of disease. There is also an increased risk of colon cancer in patients with Crohn's disease, especially in those with colitis and ileocolitis.

   e. Patients with familial polyposis, including Gardner's and Turcot's syndromes, have a nearly 100% risk of cancer by age 40. Fortunately, these are uncommon syndromes and account for less than 1% of all colon cancers. (See IV.C.)

B. Pathology

   1. Most cancers are believed to develop in adenomatous polyps (the polyp-cancer sequence). The exception to this rule is in patients with inflammatory bowel disease (IBD), in whom cancer develops in flat mucosa.

   2. Types of Polyps.

      a. Adenomatous polyps are the most common type of colon polyp. Their structure can be tubular, villous, or a combination of the two: tubulovillous. Forty percent of all cancers develop in villous adenomas, 22% develop in tubulovillous adenomas, and 5% develop in tubular adenomas. In the remaining 33%, the source of the cancer is not identifiable. Villous adenomas of the rectum or distal sigmoid may present with massive, watery diarrhea secondary to copious secretion by the polyp of fluid high in sodium, potassium, and chloride.

b. Juvenile polyps are actually hamartomatous tissue, with abundant vascular stroma containing cysts and clefts. They are called juvenile since most occur in children younger than 10 years old. They are rarely multiple. These polyps have no malignant potential but can be a source of rectal bleeding.

c. Hyperplastic polyps are also called retention polyps. They are small polyps, less than 3 mm in diameter, containing long, dilated, hyperplastic glands. They do not have malignant potential and are never a cause of bleeding or symptoms, being merely an incidental finding on colonoscopy.

d. Inflammatory polyps (pseudopolyps) are commonly found in patients with a history of colitis. They may be the only evidence that the patient had colitis of any etiology in the past, but they are not an indicator of severity of colitis. These polyps consist of mucosa with inflammatory changes and a heavy infiltrate of inflammatory cells. They thus represent islands of swollen mucosa standing out from a sea of atrophic mucosa altered by colitis. They carry no malignant potential.

3. The risk of cancer is also proportional to the size of the adenomatous polyp. A 1-cm polyp has a 1% chance of harboring cancer, whereas a polyp 1–2 cm carries a 10% risk. Polyps larger than 2 cm have a 40–50% frequency of carcinoma.

4. Staging of colorectal cancer is commonly based on the Astler and Coller modification of the Dukes classification.

a. Dukes A. Tumor limited to the mucosa (carcinoma in situ); 5-year survival 95%.

b. Dukes B. Tumor extending at least into submucosa but not involving local lymph nodes; 5-year survival 65%. A B1 lesion is defined as tumor reaching but not extending beyond the muscularis propria; a B2 lesion invades through the muscularis propria into the serosa.

c. Dukes C. Tumor involving local lymph nodes; 5-year survival 30%. A C1 lesion is defined as tumor not invading the muscularis propria; a C2 lesion is through the serosa.

    d. Dukes D. Tumor with distant metastases, usually hepatic; 5-year survival less than 5%.

  5. Prognosis also correlates with additional factors besides the depth of colon wall penetration by tumor. A poorer prognosis also is associated with lymphatic or venous invasion by tumor, poorly differentiated histology of the tumor, and greater number of lymph nodes involved.

C. Polyposis Syndromes

  1. Familial Polyposis. Autosomal dominant; multiple adenomatous polyps; 100% risk of cancer by age 40 years. Also sometimes associated with cancer of the stomach, ampulla of Vater, or small bowel.

  2. Gardner's Syndrome. Autosomal dominant; scattered adenomatous polyps, bone and cartilage tumors, sebaceous cysts; high risk of cancer. Also associated with cancers of the proximal GI tract.

  3. Turcot's syndrome. Autosomal dominant; scattered adenomatous polyps, central nervous system (CNS) tumors; high risk of cancer.

  4. Peutz-Jeghers syndrome. Autosomal dominant; multiple hamartomas associated with mucocutaneous pigmentation; increased risk of colon cancer 1–2%.

  5. Cronkhite-Canada syndrome. Multiple inflammatory polyps from mouth to anus associated with severe protein and electrolyte-losing enteropathy, onychodystrophy, and alopecia; not familial; no increased risk of cancer but often fatal nonetheless.

D. Signs and Symptoms

  1. Colon cancer should be suspected in anyone over the age of 50 years presenting with iron deficiency anemia, rectal bleeding, or a positive fecal occult blood test.

  2. Most patients develop bowel symptoms only with larger tumors and hence advanced stages of disease, which are less curable. Ninety percent of symptomatic patients have a Dukes B lesion or worse. The symptoms include change of bowel habits, new-onset constipation, or alternating diarrhea and constipation. Complaints of pencil-thin stools and tenesmus are suggestive of rectal lesions. Right colonic

lesions remain asymptomatic longer than left-sided cancers because stool is more liquid in the right colon. Patients occasionally may present with frank large bowel obstruction secondary to a constricting lesion or may present with perforation mimicking diverticulitis.

3. Physical examination in patients with colon cancer may reveal an abdominal mass due to a bulky tumor or metastases. There may be nodularity or mass on liver examination, a periumbilical mass called a Sister Mary Joseph node (not really a lymph node but metastases to the umbilical remnant), a left supraclavicular node from the thoracic duct (Virchow's node), or metastases dropped onto the rectovesical pouch that can be palpated on rectal examination (Blumer's shelf).

4. An elevated carcinoembryonic antigen (CEA) is found in many patients. This glycoprotein is not only a marker of colonic cancer but is elevated in lung and pancreatic cancers as well as inflammatory diseases such as IBD. Although the CEA test is much too insensitive and nonspecific to be useful in colon cancer screening, a high preoperative level that falls to normal after resection may allow the test to be followed postoperatively as a marker of recurrent cancer.

E. Diagnosis
1. Colorectal cancer is suspected in any patient with specific symptoms (such as change of bowel habits, new-onset constipation, or alternating diarrhea and constipation) or in asymptomatic patients with iron deficiency anemia, hematochezia, or a positive fecal occult blood test.

2. Fecal occult blood tests rely on the nature of gum guaiac, which turns blue when reduced. The developer (usually peroxide) donates hydrogen ions to the guaiac, but an enzyme is needed to perform the exchange. This enzyme is hemoglobin peroxidase in the case of a positive test. Yearly fecal blood testing is recommended by the American Cancer Society in all patients over the age of 50. A positive test carries a 20% risk of colon cancer. It is, however, an insensitive screening test for colon polyps.

3. The actual diagnosis can be made by barium enema or colonoscopy. On barium enema, the tumor may be seen as an irregular mass creating a contour defect on one wall of the colon, or it may be seen encircling and constricting a portion

of the colon, called a "napkin-ring" appearance. Colonoscopy with biopsy can also establish or confirm the diagnosis and can rule out synchronous lesions such as colon polyps, which can occur in 50% of patients, or even a second cancer, which occurs in 4% of patients.

4. Metastatic disease to the liver may be suspected in patients with an elevated alkaline phosphatase. CT scan or abdominal ultrasound can sometimes confirm the presence of metastases.

F. Therapy

1. Prevention and early detection offer the best prognosis; to this end, endoscopic surveillance combined with yearly fecal occult blood testing and digital rectal examination is advocated. Endoscopic surveillance includes sigmoidoscopy in asymptomatic patients starting at age 50, with colonoscopy reserved for patients at high risk for colon cancer. These high-risk patients include those with a history of more than 7–10 years of ulcerative colitis, previous colon polyps or cancer, previous female genital cancer, or a family history of colon cancer or polyposis syndrome.

2. Polypectomy performed endoscopically can cure a patient if cancer is still limited to the head of a pedunculated polyp. Moreover, removal of all adenomas can prevent cancer altogether.

3. Surgery is still the only curative procedure for invasive cancers. Surgery is indicated for cure in patients with cancer involving the colon wall. It is also indicated after colonoscopic polypectomy, despite complete excision, if cancer is found to be invasive in a sessile polyp, invading the stalk of a pedunculated polyp, invading the lymphatics of a polyp, or when there is a poorly differentiated histology. Cancer surgery includes removal of the tumor and the draining lymph nodes with wide margins of resection. For cancers of the cecum, ascending colon, hepatic flexure, and proximal transverse colon, a right hemicolectomy is performed. Cancers of the distal transverse colon, splenic flexure, and descending colon require a left hemicolectomy. Sigmoid cancers and some high rectal cancers may be treated with an anterior resection, but cancers of the lower rectum require abdominoperineal resection with a sigmoid colostomy.

4. Adjuvant chemotherapy or radiotherapy has been shown effective for rectal cancer.

5. Surgical palliation has a role in patients with bleeding or obstruction due to cancer. Endoscopic palliation using laser ablation of tumor is also an alternative for obstructing rectal cancers.

6. Postoperative follow-up care should include regular surveillance endoscopically and semiannual tests of CEA levels. Anastomotic recurrences are found at colonoscopy between 9–12 months postoperatively. Approximately 14% of all recurrences can be found endoscopically. The more frequent benefit of surveillance colonoscopy, however, is early detection of new metachronous lesions. An elevation of a previously normal CEA should prompt a search for recurrence. This search includes using endoscopy, chest x-ray, and abdominal CT scan. Some centers advocate second-look surgery in cases of an elevated CEA in hopes of finding a curable recurrence, although chances are slight that recurrence is curable once the CEA is elevated.

7. Solitary liver metastases are now aggressively treated in some centers with hepatic resection or intraarterial chemotherapy.

V. Pancreatic Cancer

A. Epidemiology
1. Increasing incidence; now the fourth leading cause of death from cancer, after lung, colon, and breast cancer.
2. Risk of developing pancreatic cancer is increased by smoking, alcohol abuse, and diabetes, as well as by hereditary or calcific pancreatitis. Some investigators have claimed that excessive coffee intake increases the risk of pancreatic cancer, but this hypothesis is not generally accepted.
3. This tumor carries a dismal prognosis, with the average survival 5 months from onset of initial symptoms. The 1-year survival is 10%, and 5-year survival only 1%.

B. Pathology
1. Pancreatic cancers are almost always adenocarcinomas, arising in most instances from the ductal cells. Acinar tumors do occur, although rarely. Islet cell tumors also occur (see below).

    2. Most tumors are solid, although cystadenocarcinoma occurs in some cases.

    3. Most of the tumors (70%) are located in the head of the gland, but 20% are in the body and 10% are in the tail. Since tumors in the tail do not impinge on any structures, they tend to remain silent longer than tumors in the head; patients with tumors in the tail therefore present with larger and more advanced tumors.

C. Signs and Symptoms

    1. Patients with tumors in the head of the gland often present with painless obstructive jaundice, acholic stool, dark urine, pruritus, and elevated alkaline phosphatase, due to impingement of the tumor on the common bile duct. A distended but nontender gallbladder may be palpable (Courvoisier's sign).

    2. Large tumors of the head can also compress the second portion of the duodenum, producing symptoms of gastric outlet obstruction.

    3. With obstruction of the pancreatic duct, patients may also present with symptoms of pancreatic insufficiency, e.g., weight loss, diarrhea, steatorrhea, malabsorption.

    4. Abdominal and back pain are commonly present. Although some degree of pancreatitis may be detectable at surgery, this inflammatory process is usually insignificant. The back pain is almost invariably indicative of tumor invasion of retroperitoneal structures, and it suggests inoperability.

    5. New-onset depression occurs in 5% of patients with tumors in the body or tail of the pancreas.

    6. Patients may also present with extraintestinal manifestations, e.g., polyarthritis, skin nodules of subcutaneous fat necrosis, or migratory thrombophlebitis.

    7. Patients with asymptomatic tumors in the body or tail may present with metastatic disease from the undetected primary cancer.

D. Diagnosis

    1. Tumors can be detected on CT or abdominal ultrasound.

    2. In cases of obstructive jaundice, where the diagnosis is unclear and the differential diagnosis includes choledocholithiasis, ampullary cancer, cholangiocarcinoma, and pancreatic cancer, endoscopic retrograde cholangiopancrea-

tography (ERCP) is useful in ruling out these other lesions and in demonstrating pancreatic duct obstruction. Ductal cytology performed from ERCP aspirate can help to confirm the diagnosis.

3. Angiography is able to show invasion by revealing encasement of vessels within the tumor, a sign of inoperability.

E. Therapy

1. Most therapy is palliative. Surgical palliation involves a "double bypass," which includes a choledochojejunostomy to relieve biliary obstruction and a gastroenterostomy to relieve gastric outlet obstruction. Endoscopically-placed biliary stents are also used to relieve jaundice and pruritus. The role of surgery or stenting in the patient with asymptomatic jaundice is uncertain.

2. Curative surgical resection is possible in only a few cases of pancreatic cancer limited to the head of the gland. It involves extensive resection, a radical pancreatoduodenectomy (a Whipple procedure).

F. Islet Cell Tumors

1. Pancreatic tumors originating from islet cells are distinctly different from the aggressive cancers that arise from ductal cells. These endocrine tumors are usually smaller and slower growing than ductal cell cancers. Patients come to medical attention not with outlet obstruction or jaundice but rather with symptoms attributable to the hormone secreted by the tumor. These tumors are named after the hormone they secrete.

2. Types

a. Insulinoma or β-cell tumor secretes insulin, and patients present with hypoglycemia.

b. Gastrinoma or Zollinger-Ellison syndrome is a tumor that secretes gastrin. Patients with this cancer develop hyperacidity with peptic ulceration and diarrhea.

c. Glucagonoma secretes glucagon, and patients are hyperglycemic and have a characteristic body rash.

d. VIPoma (pancreatic cholera, watery diarrhea, hypokalemia-hypochlorhydria syndrome, or Verner-Morrison syndrome) is a tumor that secretes vasoactive intestinal peptide (VIP). Patients with this cancer have massive diarrhea and electrolyte abnormalities.

e. Nonfunctioning islet cell tumor occurs rarely.
3. Ten percent of patients with islet cell tumors have other associated endocrine tumors, so-called multiple endocrine neoplasia (MEN) syndromes.
4. Once a functioning islet cell tumor is diagnosed by finding elevated serum levels of the suspected hormone, localization of the tumor may prove difficult. CT scanning, angiography, and selective venous sampling for the hormone all provide ways of discovering tumor location.
5. Surgical resection is usually curative in all of these tumors, with the exception of a gastrinoma, which generally is already metastatic at the time of diagnosis. Symptoms from metastatic gastrinoma are usually controlled with histamine-2 (H-2) antagonists.

VI. Liver Cancer

A. Epidemiology
1. Most tumors of the liver are metastatic. The most common source of metastases is the GI tract, followed by lung, breast, and ovarian cancers.
2. Worldwide, hepatocellular carcinoma (hepatoma), cancer arising from the hepatocyte, is the number one cause of death from cancer. Although it is uncommon in the United States, hepatoma is common in Africa and Asia.
3. There are many risk factors associated with hepatocellular carcinoma:
   a. Cirrhosis (found in 80% of cases).
   b. Chronic hepatitis B antigenemia.
   c. Hemochromatosis.
   d. Toxins, e.g., aflatoxin from *Aspergillus*, found on the peanut.
   e. Drugs, e.g., androgenic steroids.
   f. Thorotrast, a radiographic contrast medium no longer in use.
   g. Alcoholic liver disease.
4. Extremely poor prognosis, with average survival 3–4 months.
B. Pathology
1. The pathologist may be unable to differentiate hepatoma from intrahepatic cholangiocarcinoma, and may be forced to refer to such cases as cholangio-hepatocellular carcinoma.

2. Hepatoma metastasizes to lung, bone, and the adrenals as well as extending directly into the hepatic vein to produce Budd-Chiari syndrome.

C. Signs and Symptoms
   1. Hepatoma should be suspected in any patient with known cirrhosis who clinically deteriorates or who develops an increasing liver size on examination.
   2. Patients with hepatoma often have an abdominal mass, pain, and fever; occasionally a bruit may be heard over the hepatic mass.
   3. Patients may develop bloody ascites.
   4. Extraintestinal manifestations of erythrocytosis, hypercalcemia, or hypoglycemia may be highly symptomatic.

D. Diagnosis
   1. Abdominal ultrasound or CT scan can reveal liver masses.
   2. Metastatic disease to the liver is usually seen as multiple, uniformly sized nodules; primary liver cancer is most often a single, large mass. This rule is not hard and fast, however, since single metastatic lesions can sometimes be seen.
   3. α-Fetoprotein is elevated in 50% of cases of hepatoma, with values greater than 500 ng/ml.
   4. Gallium scanning can also be used in diagnosis; more than 90% of cases show concentration of gallium within the hepatoma.
   5. Biopsy, either percutaneous or guided by ultrasound, CT scan, or laparoscopy, can be used to confirm the diagnosis.

E. Therapy
   Most therapy is palliative, because this tumor shows little or no response to chemotherapy or radiotherapy. Surgical resection of isolated, small tumors has been successful in some cases.

VII. **Biliary Tract Cancer**

A. Epidemiology
   1. Biliary tract cancers include cancer of the gallbladder, cancer of the bile ducts (cholangiocarcinoma), and cancer of the ampulla of Vater. Gallbladder cancer is the most common, accounting for 3–6% of all GI tract cancers.
   2. They are all uncommon but are all lethal.
   3. Risk Factors.
      a. Gallbladder Cancer. Gallstones are present in 90% of

cases, although cancer develops in less than 1% of patients with gallstones. Chronic cholecystitis is believed to lead to cancer through chronic inflammation and possible infection caused by gallstones.

   b. Ampullary Cancer. Familial polyposis, Gardner's syndrome.

   c. Cholangiocarcinoma. Ulcerative colitis, sclerosing cholangitis, *Clonorchis sinensis* (liver fluke), hepatic schistosomiasis, chronic biliary tract infection (chronic cholangitis), Thorotrast exposure. Stones are not believed to be a risk factor for cholangiocarcinoma, since they are found in only one-third of patients.

B. Pathology

   1. Cholangiocarcinoma is cancer arising from the bile duct. It includes intrahepatic, extrahepatic, and intraduodenal segment (ampullary) cancers.

   2. Two-thirds of cholangiocarcinomas occur in the common bile duct or common hepatic duct. The most common sites for cholangiocarcinoma, in descending order, are the lower end of the common bile duct, the junction of the cystic duct with the common bile duct, the hepatic ducts, the cystic duct, and the ampulla of Vater. Tumor occurring at the bifurcation of the hepatic ducts is termed a Klatskin tumor.

   3. Gallbladder carcinoma is most commonly an adenocarcinoma. In 10% of cases, however, a squamous cell carcinoma is found, secondary to squamous metaplasia of the gallbladder.

   4. When tumor is widespread, the primary site, whether bile duct, ampulla, pancreas, or gallbladder, may be difficult to determine at surgery, and even pathology may reveal only a poorly differentiated adenocarcinoma.

C. Signs and Symptoms

   1. Patients with gallbladder cancer commonly present with symptoms of cholecystitis. A hard gallbladder is usually palpable.

   2. Patients with cholangiocarcinoma present with features secondary to bile duct obstruction, namely jaundice, pruritus, and cholestatic changes on liver chemistries. Ampullary tumors, because of their strategic position, usually present early, when the tumor is still small and metastatic disease

has not yet occurred. Carcinoma of the cystic duct often produces hydrops or mucocele of the gallbladder; in such cases, the tensely dilated gallbladder is usually palpable and not tender.

3. Hemobilia can occur, usually detected on a fecal occult blood test. Cancer, however, is not the most common cause of hemobilia, which is usually secondary to (in descending order): trauma, including surgery; hepatic and biliary inflammation or infection; gallstones; and finally cancer.

D. Diagnosis
   1. The diagnosis cannot be made clinically in patients presenting with obstructive jaundice. Invasive testing is necessary to differentiate pancreatic, ampullary, bile duct, gallbladder, and even duodenal cancers.
   2. CT scan and ultrasound can reveal a mass but may be unable to determine its site of origin.
   3. ERCP can be diagnostic.

E. Therapy
   1. Whipple resection can be curative in distal common bile duct and periampullary cancers. The surgery has a 10–20% mortality, but survival rates are increased in those patients selected for surgery. One-year survival rates of 84% for ampullary, 47% for pancreatic, 76% for distal common bile duct, and 94% for duodenal cancers have been reported.
   2. Surgical resection of tumors of the hepatic duct bifurcation (Klatskin tumors) is difficult. These tumors are treated with radiotherapy, including the new methods of intraoperative radiotherapy and local irradiation by means of iridium beads in a catheter that is placed in the bile duct endoscopically.
   3. Unfortunately, most tumors are not amenable to surgical resection for cure. Endoscopically placed stents or surgical bypass of the bile duct offers the best palliation.

SUGGESTED READINGS

Gastrointestinal Tumor Study Group: Prolongation of the disease-free interval in surgically treated rectal carcinoma. *N Engl J Med* 312:1465–1471, 1985.

Kobayashi K, Sugimoto T, Makino H, et al.: Screening methods for early detection of hepatocellular carcinoma. *Hepatology* 5:1100–1105, 1985.

Langer JC, Langer B, Taylor BR, et al.: Carcinoma of the extrahepatic bile ducts: results of an aggressive surgical approach. *Surgery* 98:752–759, 1985.

Minton JP, Hoehn JL, Gerber DM, et al.: Results of a 400-patient carcinoembryonic antigen second-look colorectal cancer study. *Cancer* 55:1284–1290, 1985.

Schwartz SI, Jones LS, McCune CS: Assessment of treatment of intrahepatic malignancies using chemotherapy via an implantable pump. *Ann Surg* 201:560–567, 1985.

Wilson SE, Hiatt, JR, Stable BE, et al.: Cancer of the distal esophagus and cardia: preoperative irradiation prolongs survival. *Am J Surg* 150:114–121, 1985.

Winawer SJ, Schottenfeld D, Sherlock P: *Colorectal Cancer: Prevention, Epidemiology, and Screening.* New York, Raven Press, 1980.

Chapter 19

Nutritional Assessment and Nutrient Requirements in Hospitalized Patients

Samuel Klein, M.D.[a]

I. Introduction

Malnutrition, a vague and sometimes confusing term, can be clinically defined as any impairment in whole body, organ, cellular, and/or subcellular function due to nutritional imbalances. It is associated with an increase in morbidity and mortality in hospitalized patients. Since the major function of the gastrointestinal (GI) tract is to process and absorb nutrients, patients with GI diseases are particularly susceptible to the development of nutritional abnormalities. Anorexia, dietary restrictions, malabsorption, increased GI losses, and altered nutrient requirements may all contribute to a compromised nutritional state. Nutritional intervention, therefore, can improve clinical outcome in certain patients. It is important to recognize patients at increased risk and to institute appropriate nutritional therapy when necessary.

II. Nutritional Assessment

A. Nutritional Indicators

An assessment of nutritional status is critical in evaluating a

[a]Currently at the Division of Gastroenterology, The University of Texas Medical branch, Galveston, Texas.

patient for possible nutritional support. A host of "nutritional indicators" are commonly used to measure nutritional status:
1. Body Composition.
   a. Body Weight as Percent of Ideal Body Weight (IBW). This relates individual body weight to normal population values. In general:

90–100% IBW	Normal
80–89% IBW	Mild malnutrition
70–79% IBW	Moderate malnutrition
<70% IBW	Severe malnutrition

   Misleading information, however, can sometimes be obtained when an individual's genetic body weight is not considered. For example, an individual at the upper end of normal may lose a significant degree of weight but still be within the "normal range" according to standard tables. Furthermore, body weight does not reflect body composition, so that a patient with an excess of body fluid may show normal weight yet have depleted lean body and fat masses.
   b. Percent Body Weight Loss. Unintentional weight loss of more than 1–2% body weight in 1 week, 5% body weight in 1 month, or 10% body weight in 6 months is considered to be an adverse nutritional risk factor. Loss of 40% of body weight in a normal-weight individual or 20–25% in an already malnourished individual is associated with increased morbidity and mortality. Estimation of weight loss by history, however, may be extremely inaccurate. Changes in body weight due to changes in body fluid balance may also yield misleading conclusions.
   c. Anthropometry. Triceps and subscapular skinfold thickness give an indication of body fat, while midarm muscle circumference (midarm circumference minus triceps skinfold) reflects muscle mass. Anthropometric measurements, however, suffer from inadequate reproducibility and a high degree of interobserver variability. In addition, assessment of nutritional status may vary de-

pending on the selection of reference standards. Other factors unrelated to nutrition, such as age and hydration, can also affect results.

2. Blood Tests.

a. Serum Proteins (Albumin, Prealbumin, Transferrin, Retinol-Binding Protein). Low levels of serum proteins have been found to correlate with an increase in morbidity and mortality. Factors independent of malnutrition, however, may have dramatic effects on the concentration of plasma proteins. Infection, inflammation, trauma, or surgery result in protein and fluid shifts that can dramatically alter serum concentrations. Organ damage can result in decreased blood levels due to impaired synthesis (cirrhosis) or excessive losses (protein-losing nephropathy or enteropathy), and in increased levels due to impaired metabolism (retinol-binding protein in renal failure). Furthermore, malnutrition alone may not have a significant impact on certain protein markers. Albumin levels, for example, become only slightly depressed during starvation despite a decrease in albumin synthesis. This preservation of albumin levels is due to the long half-life of albumin (20 days) and to a decrease in the rate of albumin degradation.

b. Vitamin, Macromineral, and Trace Mineral Levels. Absolute concentrations of these substances in the blood do not always reflect body stores. They can be influenced by inflammation and/or the absence of other nutrients.

3. Urine Tests.

a. Creatinine-Height Index. The excretion of creatinine in the urine is a reflection of total body muscle mass. The creatinine-height index is the ratio of the patient's creatinine excretion over 24 hours compared to expected standards. The normal standards were developed from healthy young adults and do not taken into account changes in body build and age. In addition, incomplete urine collections, dietary intake, and renal dysfunction will affect results.

b. Twenty-Four Hour Urinary Nitrogen. Nitrogen excretion can be used to estimate the degree of metabolic stress and the adequacy of exogenous protein administration.

The accuracy and significance of this test, however, may be questioned (see III.B.1).

4. Immune Competence. Malnutrition is associated with reduced immune competence.

   a. Total Lymphocyte Count. The level of lymphocyte depletion correlates the with degree of malnutrition as follows:

   1200–2000 lymphocytes/mm^3 Mild malnutrition
   800–119 lymphocytes/mm^3 Moderate malnutrition
   <800 lymphocytes/mm^3 Severe malnutrition

   Total lymphocyte count, however, is greatly affected by other factors. Certain infections may increase the lymphocyte count, and surgery may decrease the lymphocyte count.

   b. Delayed Cutaneous Hypersensitivity. Anergy to a battery of skin test antigens (*Candida*, mumps, tuberculin, streptokinase-streptodornase, *Trichophyton*) can be the result of severe malnutrition. In the hospitalized patient, skin-test responsiveness may also be affected by other factors, such as infections, medical therapy (e.g., steroids, chemotherapy), general anesthesia, surgery, trauma, burns, hemorrhage, cancer, liver disease, renal failure, and myocardial infarction.

5. Discriminant Analysis. This method can be used to determine which nutritional indicators correlate best with clinical outcome. Each of the selected indicators is given a score, and the combination reflects an overall "nutritional index." Although these calculated indices may be good predictors of outcome, the individual components are usually not independent of each other and can often be affected by factors other than nutrition.

B. Clinical Assessment

A careful history, focusing on dietary intake, weight loss, metabolic stress, and disease, in conjunction with a careful physical examination, focusing on signs of nutritional deficiencies, weight loss, and functional abilities, has been shown to be effective in predicting nutritional status and outcome. It is not clear, however, how well assessments by less skilled personnel might compare to the published reports.

C. Guidelines

All of the above nutritional indicators are imprecise and potentially misleading. In addition, many studies have failed to demonstrate that nutritional intervention consistently improves outcome, suggesting that these indicators may be markers of sicker patients rather than signs of malnutrition alone. The best approach in assessing nutritional status is probably to combine the use of several indicators tempered by clinical assessment and judgment.

III. **Nutrient Requirements**

A. Energy Needs

1. Total Daily Energy Expenditure (*TEE*). *TEE* can be divided into several components:

a. Basal Metabolic Rate (*BMR*). *BMR* is the minimal expenditure of an individual, 12–18 hours after a meal, while at complete muscular rest. *BMR* represents approximately 65% of *TEE* and 90% of the resting energy expenditure (*REE*). It is directly related to body size, age, and sex.

b. *REE* is the amount of energy expending while resting quietly several hours after meals or physical activity. It constitutes approximately 75% of the total energy expenditure (*TEE*). *REE* can be estimated using the Harris-Benedict equation (HBE). For males,

$$REE \text{ (kcal/day)} = 66.5 + (13.8 \times W) + (5 \times H) - (6.8 \times A)$$

For females,

$$REE \text{ (kcal/day)} = 655 + (9.6 \times W) + (1.8 \times H) - (4.7 \times A)$$

where *W* is weight in kg; *H* is height in cm; and *A* is age in years.

c. Thermic Effect of Muscular Work (*TEW*). *TEW* varies with activity but normally averages 15–20% of *TEE*.

d. Thermic Effect of Food (*TEF*). *TEF* varies with diet but usually accounts for 10% of *TEE*.

2. *TEE* can be calculated by multiplying the predicted *REE* by a factor to adjust for the thermic effects of food and physical activity (1.1–1.2 for patients confined to bed, 1.2–1.3 for patients allowed out of bed), and by a metabolic factor related to the severity of the particular disease state (1.0–1.6).

Table 19.1.
Metabolic Factors for Use in Calculating Total Daily Energy Expenditure

Disease State	Metabolic Factor
Elective surgery	1.0–1.2
Fever	1.0+0.13 per °C
Inflammatory bowel disease	1.0–1.2
Sepsis, peritonitis	1.2–1.6

Metabolic factors for various disease states are shown in Table 19.1.

For example, the energy requirements of a 25-year-old, 70-kg, 175-cm male patient admitted to the hospital with an exacerbation of Crohn's disease would be:

$$REE = 66.5 + (13.8 \times 70) + (5 \times 175) - (6.8 \times 25) = 1738 \text{ kcal/day}$$
$$TEE = REE \times \text{activity factor} \times \text{stress factor}$$
$$TEE = 1738 \times 1.2 \times 1.2 = 2503 \text{ kcal/day}$$

B. Macronutrients
1. Protein. Protein is essential for vital structures and functions. One important goal of nutritional therapy is to supply enough exogenous protein to meet body requirements.
   a. Nitrogen Balance. The adequacy of protein intake can be estimated by using nitrogen as a protein marker. Nitrogen balance, therefore, reflects protein balance:

   Nitrogen balance = Nitrogen in − nitrogen out

   where nitrogen in (grams) = protein intake (grams)/6.25 (since protein contains approximately 16% nitrogen), and nitrogen out (grams) = urinary nitrogen and nitrogen losses from other minor routes (e.g., feces, sweat, respiration). Several factors, however, affect the interpretation of nitrogen balance data. There may be an "apparent" retention of nitrogen in normal individuals consuming protein above the maintenance requirements. In addition, estimates of daily nitrogen losses from unquantified sources may be incorrect in many patients. Normal renal function and complete urine collections are also necessary for the accuracy of the calculations.
   b. Protein Requirements. Several factors influence protein requirements:

      i. The amount of nonprotein calories in the diet. Protein requirements increase when caloric intake does not meet energy needs. The magnitude of this increase is directly proportional to the decrease in energy supply. Conversely, at any level of suboptimal protein intake, nitrogen balance can be improved by increasing energy intake.

     ii. The metabolic state of the patient. Catabolic illness, which increases metabolic rate, also increases protein needs. The amount of protein needed to maintain nitrogen balance becomes progressively higher as metabolic rate increases, even when energy intake meets total energy requirements. Therefore, while the calorie:nitrogen ratio needed to maintain nitrogen balance is approximately 300:1 in normal subjects, it decreases to 150:1 during severe illness and stress.

    iii. The amino acid composition of the protein source. The utilization of protein and amino acids is determined, in part, by the availability of adequate amounts of essential amino acids in the protein source. Inadequate amounts of any of the essential amino acids will result in inefficient utilization. In general, approximately 15–20% of total protein needs are required to be in the form of essential amino acids in normal adults. Since the body can conserve essential amino acids when they are in limited supply, the amino acid composition of the protein source is usually not important except in cases where exceptionally poor quality protein is used.

    iv. Guidelines for daily protein requirements in adult patients are shown in Table 19.2.

2. Carbohydrate.
   a. Calorie Source. Carbohydrate, usually in the form of glucose, is the least expensive and most abundant source of energy, providing 4 kcal/gram.
   b. Metabolic Implications. The major beneficial effect of carbohydrate is its role in inhibiting the breakdown of body protein. This is accomplished by its effects on endogenous glucose production and glucose oxidation.
      i. Gluconeogenesis. Several tissues require glucose as a fuel source: red blood cells, white blood cells, bone

Table 19.2.
Guidelines for Daily Protein Requirements in Adult Patients

Metabolic State	Requirement (g/kg/day)
Normal	0.5
Metabolic "stress"	0.8–2.0
Hemodialysis	1.2
Peritoneal dialysis	1.5

marrow, renal medulla, and peripheral nerve utilize about 40 grams/day. Other tissues prefer glucose when it is available: the brain utilizes about 120 grams/day. Since the body can synthesize glucose from amino acids and glycerol, there is no absolute dietary requirement for carbohydrate. Provision of adequate glucose calories, however, can minimize the breakdown of muscle protein by lowering the rate of gluconeogenesis.

ii. Glucose Oxidation. The oxidation of glucose spares the oxidation of amino acids. In general, less than 50% of glucose taken up by cells is oxidized for fuel. The oxidation of exogenous glucose is proportional to the amount of glucose given, until a certain threshold level is reached. Infusing more than 7 mg/kg/ minute (approximately 2800 kcal/day) in stable postoperative patients does not result in any further increases in fuel utilization, but it does increase lipogenesis, metabolic rate, CO_2 production, and water production.

3. Fat.

a. Calorie Source.

i. Long-Chain Triglycerides (LCTs). LCTs provide approximately 9 kcal/gram. They are as efficacious as carbohydrate in maintaining nitrogen balance in normal or depleted subjects, provided 150–200 grams of carbohydrate is given daily. The utilization of exogenous fat as a fuel source in hypermetabolic states, such as sepsis and burns, however, may not be efficient. LCTs require adequate digestive and absorptive processes for normal assimilation. Providing 30–40% of total calories as fat is recommended for a normal diet, but this figure may need modification in certain disease states, such as the hyperlipidemias.

ii. Medium-Chain Triglycerides (MCTs). MCTs contain fatty acids of 6–12 carbon lengths. They require little or no pancreatic lipase activity or bile salts for absorption, and they travel directly into the portal system without incorporation into chylomicrons. Theoretically, they provide 8.3 kcal/gram (115 kcal/tablespoon), but approximately 20% of ingested MCTs are oxidized to dicarboxylic acids. Since dicarboxylic acids cannot be utilized as fuel, the effective caloric content of MCTs is approximately 7.1 kcal/gram (92 kcal/tablespoon). Up to 4 tablespoons (370 kcal) daily is usually well tolerated.

b. Essential Fatty Acid (EFA) Source. Linoleic and linolenic acid cannot by synthesized by mammals and must be provided exogenously. Linoleic acid should constitute at least 2% and linolenic acid at least 0.5% of the daily caloric intake to prevent the occurrence of EFA deficiency.

C. Fluids

Water is essential to replace insensible, GI, and urinary losses. In general, 1 ml per kcal of energy intake is required for adults, but this figure may vary greatly depending on the clinical situation.

D. Macrominerals

Guidelines for daily macromineral requirements are shown in Table 19.3.

E. Trace Minerals

Guidelines for daily trace mineral requirements are shown in Table 19.4.

F. Vitamins

Guidelines for daily vitamin requirements are shown in Table 19.5.

G. Special Considerations in Patients with GI Tract Losses

GI suction, fistulas, or diarrhea can result in large losses of electrolytes, requiring specific replacement therapy. Although direct measurement of excreted fluids is the most accurate method of determining these losses, Table 19.6 provides guidelines for estimating electrolyte concentrations in GI tract secretions.

Table 19.3.
Guidelines for Daily Macromineral Requirements[a]

Mineral	1 Milliequivalent (mg)	Requirement	
		Enteral	Parenteral (mg)
Sodium	23	0.5–5 g	45–150
Potassium	39	2–5 g	20–150
Chloride	35.4	1–5 g	45–150
Magnesium	12	300–400 mg	10–30
Calcium	20	800–1200 mg	10–30
Phosphorus	15.5	800–1200 mg	20–60

[a]Amounts may vary depending on the type of illness present.

Table 19.4.
Guidelines for Daily Trace Mineral Requirements[a]

Mineral	Requirement	
	Enteral	Parenteral
Chromium	30–200µg	10–20 µg
Copper[b,c]	2 mg	0.3 mg
Iodine	150 µg	70–140 µg
Manganese[c]	1.5 mg	0.2–0.8 mg
Selenium	500–200 µg	20–40 µg
Zinc[b]	15 mg	2.5–4 mg
Fluoride	1.5–4 mg	0.07–0.5 mg

[a]The requirements for arsenic, cadmium, cobalt, molybdenum, nickel, silicon, and vanadium in human nutrition are not known.
[b]Increased requirements with diarrheal diseases.
[c]Decreased requirements in cholestatic liver disease.

Table 19.5.
Guidelines for Daily Vitamin Requirements

	Requirement	
	Enteral	Parenteral
Vitamin A (Retinol)	5000 IU	3300 IU
Vitamin D (Ergocalciferol)	400 IU	200 IU
Vitamin E (Alpha tocopherol)	10–15 IU	10 IU
Vitamin K (Phylloquinone)	50–100 µg	100 µg
Vitamin B$_1$ (Thiamin)	1–1.5 mg	3 mg

Table 19.5. (continued)
Guidelines for Daily Vitamin Requirements

	Requirement	
	Enteral	Parenteral
Vitamin B$_2$ (Riboflavin)	1.1–1.8 mg	3.6 mg
Vitamin B$_3$ (Pantothenic acid)	5–10 mg	15 mg
Vitamin B$_5$ (Niacin)	12–20 mg	40 mg
Vitamin B$_6$ (Pyrodoxine)	1–2mg	4 mg
Vitamin B$_7$ (Biotin)	100–200 µg	60 µg
Vitamin B$_9$ (Folic acid)	400 µg	400 µg
Vitamin B$_{12}$ (Cobalamin)	3 µg	5 µg
Vitamin C (Ascorbic acid)	60 mg	100 mg

Table 19.6.
Guidelines for Estimating Electrolyte Concentration in GI Tract Secretions

	NA (mEq/L)	K (mEq/L)	Cl (mEq/L)	HCO$_3$ (mEq/L)
Gastric fluid	65	10	100	—
Biliary fistula	150	4	100	35
Pancreatic fistula	150	7	80	75
Duodenal fluid	90	15	90	15
Mid-small bowel fluid	140	6	100	20
Terminal ileum fluid	140	8	60	70
Diarrhea	40	90	15	30

SUGGESTED READINGS

Baker JP, Detsky AS, Wesson DE, et al.: Nutritional assessment: a comparison of clinical judgement and objective measurements. *N Engl J Med* 306:969–972, 1982.

Bernard MA, Jacobs DO, Rombeau JL: *Nutritional and Metabolic Support of Hospitalized Patients.* Philadelphia, WB Saunders, 1986.

Blackburn GL, Bistrian BR, Maini BS, Schlamm HT, Smith MF: Nutritional and metabolic assessment of the hospitalized patient. *J Parenter Enteral Nutr* 1:11–22, 1977.

Buzby GP, Mullen JL, Matthews DC, Hobbs CL, Rosato EF: Prognostic nutritional index in gastrointestinal surgery. *Am J Surg* 139:160–167, 1980.

Goodhart RS, Shils ME: *Modern Nutrition in Health and Disease.* Philadelphia, Lea & Febiger, 1980.

Rombeau JL, Caldwell MD: *Clinical Nutrition: Enteral and Tube Feeding,* vol 1. Philadelphia, WB Saunders, 1984.

Rombeau JL, Caldwell MD: *Clinical Nutrition: Parenteral Nutrition,* vol 2. Philadelphia, WB Saunders, 1986.

Chapter 20

Enteral and Parenteral Nutrition in Hospitalized Patients

Samuel Klein, M.D.[a]

I. Enteral Nutrition

  A. Principles

    1. Whenever possible, the gastrointestinal (GI) tract should be the site used for nutritional support.

    2. Enteral feeding is less expensive, safer, and more physiologic than parenteral nutrition.

    3. Luminal nutrients are required to maintain the integrity of the GI tract. Mucosal atrophy, decreased brush border enzyme activity, impaired function of the gut-associated immune system, and increased translocation of bacteria into the systemic circulation may occur with bowel rest.

  B. Feeding Regimens

    1. Hospital Diets.

      a. Clear Liquids. This diet consists of nondairy foods that are liquid at room temperature, such as broths, juices, coffee, tea, gelatin, and ices. It is usually used to prevent dehydration and minimize dietary residue prior to GI procedures or to assess the condition of the gastrointesti-

[a]Currently at the Division of Gastroenterology, The University of Texas Medical Branch, Galveston, Texas.

nal tract before instituting a more rigorous feeding trial. The clear liquid diet does not provide adequate calories, protein, vitamins, or minerals.

b. Full Liquids. This diet consists of foods that liquify at room temperature, including milk products such as milk, custards, juices, milkshakes, and ice cream. It is usually used in the transition from clear liquids to solid foods. With appropriate supplements, the full liquid diet can be nutritionally adequate. The large amount of lactose in this diet, however, prohibits its use in many patients.

c. Low-Residue, Low-Fiber Diet. This diet restricts fiber and other foods that increase stool volume, such as prune juice, but includes cooked vegetables and fruits, and tender meats. This diet may be efficacious in patients with partial intestinal obstruction and during exacerbations of inflammatory bowel disease or diverticulitis.

d. High-Fiber Diet. This diet increases total daily fiber intake to 15 or more grams/day by increasing the intake of whole grains and raw fruit and vegetables. It is effective in increasing the volume and weight of stool and decreasing intraluminal colonic pressure.

e. Low-Fat Diet. This diet restricts all forms of fat to less than 50 grams/day. It is often useful in patients with impaired fat digestion/absorption due to causes such as pancreatic insufficiency or ileal resection.

f. Low-Sodium Diet. This diet restricts sodium to 500–2000 mg/day. In comparison, the average American diet contains 6000 mg of sodium daily. The low-sodium diet is useful in promoting diuresis in patients with cirrhosis, congestive heart failure, and renal failure when sodium and water retention occur.

2. Food Supplements. These can be added as needed to enhance the patient's routine diet or feeding formula.

a. Protein Modules. These contain either intact protein, hydrolyzed protein, or crystalline amino acids. They are relatively insoluble, particularly when in powder form. The smaller the size of the protein particle, the greater the cost and osmolality, and the worse the palatability of the formula. Crystalline amino acids, therefore, are usually administered by tube.

    b. Carbohydrate Modules. These are usually in the form of glucose or glucose polymers. The smaller the polymer, the greater its osmolality and sweetness. In general, carbohydrate modules are relatively inexpensive and water-soluble, readily mixing with other formulas or foods.

    c. Fat Modules. These include formulas consisting of long-chain fats (butter fat, vegetable oils, and fat emulsions) and formulas consisting of medium-chain triglycerides. They have a high caloric density and contribute little to osmolality.

3. Polymeric Formulas. These formulas can provide adequate calories, protein, essential fatty acids (EFAs), vitamins, and minerals if given in appropriate quantities. The specific requirements of the clinical situation, tolerance, and taste preference in patients being fed orally dictate which formula is used in each case.

    a. Blenderized Diets. These are pureed formulas containing beef and/or milk as a protein source, cereal, fruits and/or vegetables as a carbohydrate source, and corn or soy oil as a fat source. They are useful in preventing constipation in patients requiring chronic enteral feeding. A large-bore feeding tube is required because of their poor palatability and high viscosity. These diets are high in residue, contain 1 kcal/ml, and have an osmolality in the range of 300–450 mOsm.

    b. Milk-Based Formulas. These tend to be more palatable than other formulas. They consist of intact proteins, mono-, di- and polysaccharides and long-chain fats and are useful in lactose-tolerant patients. They generally contain more protein and lactose than other formulas, are high in residue, contain 1 kcal/ml, and have an osmolality of 500–700 mOsm.

    c. Lactose-Free Formulas. These contain intact proteins, di- and oligosaccharides, and long-chain and medium-chain fats. They have a low viscosity (making them ideal for tube feeding), are low in residue, provide 1 kcal/ml, and have an osmolality in the range of 300–450 mOsm.

4. Predigested Formulas. These elemental and peptide formulas require minimal digestive function of the GI tract for absorption and may be useful in patients with severe pan-

creatic exocrine insufficiency or active Crohn's disease. They contain protein in the form of amino acids and/or small peptides, carbohydrate as simple glucose oligosaccharides, and a minimal amount of fat as long-chain and/or medium-chain triglycerides. Protein in the form of di- and tri-peptides is absorbed more efficiently than free amino acids or longer peptides. Because of problems with palatability, these formulas are usually administered by feeding tube. They are expensive, low in residue, contain 1 kcal/ml, and are hyperosmolar (approximately 450–800 mOsm).

5. Specialty Formulas. These are designed for patients with specific nutritional needs. The benefit of these formulas over the less expensive standard solutions requires further documentation before their routine use can be recommended.

   a. Essential Amino Acid Formula. This formula has been recommended for patients with renal failure. It contains essential amino acids only, mono- and disaccharides, and long-chain fats. It does not contain vitamins or minerals, with the exception of negligible amounts of sodium and potassium. It provides 2 kcal/ml and is hyperosmolar (850 mOsm).

   b. Branched-Chain Amino Acid-Enriched Formula. This formula has been recommended in patients with hepatic encephalopathy, severe trauma, and sepsis. It contains a protein source high in branched-chain and low in aromatic amino acids, and also contains mono- and disaccharides and long-chain fats. It does not have vitamins or minerals except for negligible amounts of sodium, contains 1.7 kcal/ml, and is hyperosmolar (900 mOsm).

   c. Calorie-Dense Formulas. These have been recommended in patients who are hypermetabolic or require fluid restriction. They contain 1.5–2.0 kcal/ml and have a high osmolality (approximately 600 mOsm).

   d. High-Fat Formula. This has been recommended for patients with respiratory insufficiency, since the high fat content (55% of calories) and low carbohydrate content (28% of calories) reduces the production of carbon dioxide. It contains 1.5 kcal/ml and 490 mOsm/kg.

6. Oral Rehydration Therapy. By taking advantage of normal mucosal absorptive processes, it is possible to replace water

and salt losses orally in many patients who have severe diarrhea. The active absorption of glucose or amino acids usually remains intact in many diarrheal diseases and involves a common carrier with sodium. Ingestion of solutions containing glucose (or amino acids) and sodium results in active sodium transport and passive water absorption through the intestinal mucosa; cereal starches may provide the same absorptive benefits at a lower osmolar cost.

C. Tube Feeding
  1. Techniques.
    a. Feeding Sites. Nasogastric, nasoduodenal, nasojejunal, gastrostomy, jejunostomy, pharyngostomy, and esophagostomy tubes can all be used for feeding. Feeding into the stomach is usually preferable, since tolerance is better, especially when hyperosmolar or bolus feedings are used. Patients with a history of aspiration, pulmonary disease, delayed gastric emptying, or abnormal mental/neurologic status may have fewer serious complications with small intestinal feedings, since the pyloric sphincter provides another barrier to reflux of intestinal contents.
    b. Delivery Schedule.
      i. Bolus Feeding. This resembles normal feeding patterns and is useful in alert patients with normal gastric emptying. In other patients, however, it may result in an increased incidence of aspiration.
      ii. Continuous Feeding. Tolerance is usually better with a continuous infusion of nutrients, resulting in the ability to provide more daily calories.
    c. Initiating Feedings. "Starter regimens," in which initial enteral feedings are diluted to hypoosmolar concentrations, do not improve patient tolerance but do decrease the amount of nutrients given. Tube feedings can be started with full-strength isoosmolar formulas at low infusion rates (e.g., 50 ml/hour) and can be increased by 25–30 ml/hour per day as tolerated until the desired amount is reached.
    d. Complications.
      i. Mechanical. Nasopharyngeal and esophageal irritation, tube clogging, and nasotracheal intubation. Tube

enterostomies may leak, excoriate the skin, and result in severe wound infections.
ii. Metabolic. Volume overload, dehydration, glucose and electrolyte abnormalities.
iii. GI. Abdominal discomfort, diarrhea, and pulmonary aspiration.

II. Parenteral Nutrition

A. Total Parenteral Nutrition (TPN)
1. Indications. Identifying patients in whom TPN will reduce morbidity and mortality is difficult because of the paucity of well-designed, prospective, randomized clinical trials. The following is a list of conditions in which clinical trials or clinical experience suggest a beneficial effect of TPN. This list is based on the current available literature and may need modification based on future clinical trials.
   a. Conditions involving the adverse effects of starvation, such as:
      i. "Short bowel" syndrome.
      ii. Intestinal obstruction/pseudoobstruction.
      iii. Growth retardation in children.
      iv. Hyperemesis gravidarum.
   b. Conditions involving increased metabolic demands, such as:
      i. Major burns.
      ii. Head injury.
   c. Conditions that may benefit from GI "rest," such as:
      i. Crohn's disease.
      ii. Pancreatitis.
      iii. GI fistulas.
   d. Cancer.
      i. Preoperatively for upper GI tract cancers.
      ii. Bone marrow transplant.
   e. Organ failure.
      i. Acute renal failure.
      ii. Hepatic encephalopathy.
2. Technique.
   a. Percutaneous cannulation of a large-bore, high-flow vessel (subclavian vein or superior vena cava) allows for the relatively safe infusion of hyperosmolar (approximately

1500 mOsm for usual TPN), calorie-dense solutions.
  b. Careful monitoring once TPN has been instituted is essential to prevent unnecessary complications:
   i. Clinical Assessment. Body temperature, heart rate, and blood pressure should be checked every 8 hours. Body weight and fluid intake and output should be recorded daily. Physical examinations should be performed daily to assess body fluid status and to seek evidence of infection or nutritional deficiencies. Dressing changes and inspection of the catheter insertion site should be performed 2 or 3 times per week.
   ii. Laboratory Tests. Plasma glucose, Na, K, Cl, HCO_3, Mg, Ca, PO_4, blood urea nitrogen (BUN), and creatinine should be evaluated daily after initiating TPN until values are stable and then followed every 3–4 days. Serum triglycerides should be checked before and at least once during the infusion of lipid emulsions. Liver function tests should be obtained every 1–2 weeks.
3. Parenteral Solutions.
  a. Protein Source.
   i. Standard Solutions. Crystalline amino acids are the most commonly used source of nitrogen in parenteral nutrition. They are provided commercially in concentrations between 3 and 10% and contain 40–50% essential and 50–60% nonessential amino acids. Although the products differ in their individual amino acid and electrolyte profiles, it is not known whether these variations are clinically important.
   ii. Specialty Formulas.
    a. High branched-chain amino acid solutions. These solutions have been advocated for use in patients with hepatic encephalopathy and sepsis, but further studies are needed before firm recommendations can be made. In these special formulas, the branched-chain amino acids contribute approximately 35–45% of the total amino acids, whereas in standard formulas they constitute only about 20% of the total.

    b. High essential amino acid solutions. These have been recommended for patients with renal failure, but their use remains controversial. These formulas contain all of the essential amino acids and histidine and variable amounts of other nonessential amino acids.

b. Carbohydrate Source.

  i. Dextrose. Dextrose (glucose) is the least expensive and most commonly used intravenous energy source. Commercially made formulas are available in concentrations from 5 to 70%. The dextrose in intravenous solutions is hydrated, so that each gram of dextrose monohydrate provides only 3.4 kcal. Solutions with high concentrations of dextrose, usually 25–35%, are needed to supply adequate calories in TPN.

  ii. Other carbohydrates, such as fructose, and xylitol, cannot be recommended for routine use at the present time.

c. Fat Source. Lipid emulsions. Fat emulsions are used to supply fat intravenously. They contain soybean or safflower oil triglycerides, egg yolk phospholipids as an emulsifying agent, and glycerin to achieve isotonicity with plasma. The emulsified particles are approximately the same size as chylomicrons (0.5 µm) and are metabolized in a similar fashion. They contain approximately 50–70% linoleic acid and 5–10% linolenic acid, depending on the source of fat, and can be administered as a 10% (1.1 kcal/ml) or 20% (2.0 kcal/ml) solution. To minimize complications, no more than 3 grams/kg/day should be infused. Although it is generally recommended that the maximum amount of fat be limited to 60% of total calories, intravenous fat emulsions have been reported to supply up to 83% of total calories without adverse effects. Since calories provided from lipid emulsions are approximately six times the cost of intravenous glucose, glucose should be the major source of energy. Providing 500–1000 kcal/week as intravenous lipids is adequate to prevent EFA deficiency. In special circumstances, such as glucose intolerance, fluid overload, and respiratory insufficiency, increasing the amount of fat calories, and thereby decreasing the glucose, water, and CO_2 load, may be beneficial.

4. Compatible Medications. The addition of medications to the TPN solution can simplify patient management, especially when fluid overload and adequate venous access are problems. The following is a list of commonly used medications that are usually compatible with TPN solutions:

Aminophylline
Cimetidine
Digoxin
Heparin
Hydrocortisone
Insulin
Methyldopa
Methylprednisolone
Metoclopramide
Ranitidine

5. Complications.
   a. Catheter-Related. Trauma, thrombosis, embolus, and infection.
   b. Metabolic. Fluid imbalance, electrolyte disturbances, glucose abnormalities, specific nutrient deficiencies/excesses, and bone disease.
   c. GI Diseases.
      i. Liver Disease.
         a. Mild liver function test abnormalities with elevated transaminases and alkaline phosphatase sometimes occur but are probably not clinically significant.
         b. Fatty liver due to carbohydrate overload, decreased EFAs, or malnutrition may occur.
         c. Cholestasis may occur—usually due to sepsis and not TPN.
         d. Chronic liver disease has been reported to occur in up to 5% of patients on long-term TPN. Many of these patients had preexisting liver disease.
      ii. Gallbladder Disease. This problem is probably secondary to decreased gallbladder emptying and in-

creased bile lithogenicity.

    a. Sludge occurs in the gallbladder in almost all patients after 6 weeks of TPN.

    b. Gallstones usually occur in those patients who have already developed gallbladder sludge.

    c. Acalculous cholecystitis may occur.

  iii. Villous and Pancreatic Atrophy. These lesions are due to the lack of luminal nutrients and they resolve rapidly after refeeding.

B. Peripheral Parenteral Nutrition (PPN)

  1. Indications. Peripheral veins can be used to administer nutrients in patients who require parenteral nutrition when catheterization of a central vein is not possible or desirable. Since PPN is usually hypocaloric relative to energy needs, and since venous access becomes limited in most patients after several days, PPN is not a means of providing prolonged nutritional support.

  2. Technique.

    a. Solutions.

      i. Protein. Amino acids are usually given in a 2.5–5% concentration providing 25–50 grams of protein per liter.

     ii. Carbohydrate. Dextrose is usually given in a 5–10% concentration providing 170–340 kcal/L.

    iii. Fat. Lipid emulsions are critical in providing a rich caloric source. The amount should be limited to a maximum of 2–3 grams/kg per day.

    b. Daily Nutrient Infusion. The large volumes of fluid needed to supply adequate calories are prohibitive in many patients. For example, for PPN to provide 1500 kcal (66% from fat) and 100 grams of protein would require approximately 3 liters of a combined 3.5% amino acid and 5% dextrose solution plus 500 cc of a 20% lipid emulsion.

  3. Complications.

    a. Thrombophlebitis. The frequency of catheterization site thrombophlebitis is a limiting factor in the use of PPN. This complication is related to the osmolality of the intravenous solutions. The addition of standard electrolytes to the solution described in 2.b, above results in a final osmolality of approximately 900 mOsm. Small amounts of heparin (500–3000 units/L) and/or cortisol (5 mg/L) may decrease the incidence of phlebitis. Simultaneous infusion of an isotonic lipid emulsion into the same vein will decrease the osmolality of the amino acid-dextrose mixture entering the vein.

b. Metabolic complications. These are usually related to an inability to tolerate the large volume of fluid or the large quantity of lipids that are infused with PPN.

SUGGESTED READINGS

Bernard MA, Jacobs DO, Rombeau JL: *Nutritional and Metabolic Support of Hospitalized Patients.* Philadelphia, WB Saunders, 1986.

Goodhart RS, Shils ME: *Modern Nutrition in Health and Disease.* Philadelphia, Lea & Febiger, 1980.

Law DH: Current concepts in nutrition: total parenteral nutrition. *N Engl J Med* 297:1104–1107, 1977.

Michel L, Serrano A, Malt RA: Current concepts: nutritional support of hospitalized patients. *N Engl J Med* 304:1147–1152, 1981.

Rombeau JL, Caldwell MD: *Clinical Nutrition: Enteral and Tube Feeding,* vol 1. Philadelphia, WB Saunders, 1986.

Rombeau JL, Caldwell MD: *Clinical Nutrition: Enteral and Tube Feeding,* vol 2. Philadelphia, WB Saunders, 1986.

Chapter 21

Diagnostic and Therapeutic Endoscopy

Jerome D. Waye, M.D.

I. **Esophagogastroduodenoscopy (EGD)/Upper Intestinal Endoscopy**

A. Description

Upper intestinal endoscopy is performed with flexible instruments passed through the cricopharynx under direct vision in the patient who has received mild sedation, usually with meperidine and a benzodiazepine. A topical anesthetic may be used to anesthetize the posterior pharynx. The procedure is well tolerated, with modern instruments being less than 10 mm in diameter. Direct visualization of the entire esophagus, stomach, and duodenum (to the junction of the second and third portions) can be accomplished easily, and targeted biopsies may be obtained at any site.

B. Endoscopy and X-Ray

Primary endoscopy is becoming more common without preceding upper gastrointestinal (GI) x-ray series. The small-caliber instruments are well tolerated with a low incidence of risk. The correct technique of introducing the gastroscope under direct vision makes primary endoscopy safe.

C. Indications
1. Upper abdominal distress that has not responded to a 4- to 6-week trial of symptomatic therapy.
2. Upper abdominal distress associated with a short history of signs or symptoms suggesting significant associated disease (vomiting, anorexia, weight loss, etc.).
3. Dysphagia or odynophagia.
4. Esophageal reflux symptoms that persist despite appropriate therapy.
5. Persistent unexplained vomiting.
6. Upper GI x-ray findings of:
   a. Any lesion that requires biopsy for proper diagnosis.
   b. Suspicion of cancer in a gastric ulcer.
   c. Evidence of stricture or obstruction.
7. GI bleeding.
   a. EGD should be the first diagnostic modality in most actively bleeding patients.
   b. For presumed chronic blood loss and iron deficiency anemia when investigation of large bowel is negative.
8. Therapeutic endoscopy.
   a. Treatment of bleeding lesions.
   b. Removal of foreign bodies.
   c. Sclerotherapy for esophageal varices.
   d. Dilatation of strictures in the upper intestinal tract.
D. Therapeutic Upper Intestinal Endoscopy
1. Dilatation of strictures may be accomplished with a balloon placed through the endoscope and inflated using hydrostatic pressure. This method is effective and is associated with a low morbidity. Rubber dilators, called bougies, may be passed through the esophagus. Bougies are available in various sizes, up to a diameter of approximately 2.0 cm. Fluoroscopy is usually not required for balloons passed through the instrument (under direct vision), or for dilatation with rubber bougies. However, plastic bougies and other dilating probes are usually passed over a guide wire under fluoroscopic control. Patients may require heavier sedation for this type of therapeutic endoscopy than for diagnostic endoscopy.
2. Esophageal varices may be injected with a variety of sclerosant solutions. There is controversy as to whether injections

should be intravariceal or paravariceal, but either seems to work well. Eradication of varices requires, on the average, five sclerotherapy sessions, with multiple injections of sclerosant given during each session.

3. Most foreign bodies may successfully be removed with the flexible instruments. Foreign bodies in the esophagus or stomach (i.e., quarters, batteries, or even impacted food) are usually retrieved by pulling the foreign body out with the endoscope after having captured the object with a snare device/grasping forceps.

4. GI bleeding may be treated with a variety of methods, including laser fibers passed through the endoscope (an expensive, but effective, method for hemostasis), or direct contact heater probes. Hemostatic injections may be made into or around the bleeding vessel with either a large volume of saline/epinephrine solutions, or a small volume of absolute alcohol, both of which are relatively inexpensive and effective for therapy of acute bleeding.

E. Indications for Follow-up EGD
 1. Biopsy surveillance of patients with Barrett's esophagus.
 2. Follow-up of large indeterminate ulcers.
 3. Follow-up of patients having a previous gastric polypectomy for adenoma.

F. Situations in Which Periodic EGD Is Usually Not Indicated
 1. Surveillance of healed, benign disease such as gastric or duodenal ulcer or repeated dilatations of benign esophageal strictures.
 2. Cancer surveillance in patients with pernicious anemia, treated achalasia, or prior gastric resection.

G. Preparation for Endoscopy
The patient should be kept NPO for 6 hours.

H. Contraindications for EGD
Contraindications for EGD include recent myocardial infarction or an acute abdomen.

I. Complications of EGD
 1. Complications of upper intestinal endoscopy include medication reactions, aspiration, and cardiovascular complications such as arrhythmia and hypotension.
 2. Complications related to instrumentation include perforation of the esophagus or stomach at a rate of 1 in 10,000 with

diagnostic procedures. The incidence of complications increases when therapeutic maneuvers are performed. Bleeding may occur following removal of gastric polyps.

II. Colonoscopy

A. Description

Total colonoscopy can be performed in over 90% of patients with a standard 6-foot-long flexible endoscope. Colonoscopy is frequently used as a primary diagnostic modality, without a preceding barium enema x-ray examination, in patients suspected of having structural colon disease. Most examinations are performed with intravenous sedation (meperidine and a benzodiazepine) and are well tolerated. The procedure is usually performed with the patient in the left lateral decubitus position. Fluoroscopy is rarely utilized for the performance of colonoscopy.

B. Indications

1. Evaluation of an abnormality on the barium enema x-ray examination.
2. Evaluation of unexplained GI bleeding such as:
   a. Hematochezia.
   b. Melena with a negative upper GI investigation.
   c. Unexplained fecal occult blood.
   d. Unexplained iron deficiency anemia.
3. Surveillance for colon neoplasia.
   a. In patients who have had a previous colon cancer.
   b. In patients with previous colon polyps.
   c. In patients with a family history of colon cancer.
   d. In patients with chronic ulcerative colitis of more than 8 years duration, colonoscopy is indicated every 1–2 years, with multiple biopsies for detection of cancer and dysplasia.
4. Chronic colonic inflammatory bowel disease, if more precise diagnosis or determination of the extent of activity of disease will influence management.
5. Therapeutic colonoscopy for reasons such as control of bleeding, colonic decompression, removal of colon polyps, removal of foreign bodies, dilatation of strictures.
6. Unexplained chronic diarrhea.

C. Contraindications for Colonoscopy
   1. Fulminant colitis.
   2. Possible perforated viscus.
   3. Acute, severe diverticulitis.
D. Preparation for Endoscopy
   A clean colon is required for endoscopy. Therefore, one of the following preparatory routines should be used.
   1. Twenty-four to forty-eight hours of full liquid diet, 2 oz. castor oil or 10 oz. magnesium citrate the night before the examination, and a tap water enema 3 hours and again 2 hours before the examination.
   2. Electrolyte solution, an iso-osmolar solution of salts and polyethylene glycol, which flushes the intestinal tract without inducing salt or water overload. Patient should drink 1 gallon of fluid over a 3-hour period on the evening prior to the exam or 6 hours before colonoscopy.
      a. Patients should avoid food or liquids within 3 hours of drinking the solution because sodium and fluid absorption, which are nil with the electrolyte preparation alone, are stimulated by any glucose-containing substance.
E. Complications
   1. Medication reactions, comprising such cardiovascular complications as arrhythmia, and hypotension.
   2 Perforation occurs in 1 case in 1000, but bleeding following a polypectomy may occur in as many as 3% of cases.

III. **Flexible Sigmoidoscopy (FS)**

   A. Description
   The examination with a 30-cm or 60-cm flexible instrument permits visualization of the rectum and a variable portion of the sigmoid and descending colon. It is performed with the patient in the left lateral decubitus position. Sedation is generally not employed.
   B. Indications
   1. Screening of asymptomatic patients at risk for colon neoplasia.
   2. Evaluation of suspected distal colonic disease when there is no indication for colonoscopy.
   3. Evaluation of the colon in conjunction with barium enema.

C. Recommendations
For neoplasia detection, the American Cancer Society recommends two annual examinations one year apart at age 50 years, and, if both are negative, an examination every 3 years subsequently.

D. Contraindications
1. Fulminant colitis.
2. Severe, acute diverticulitis.
3. Peritonitis.

E. Situations in Which FS is Generally Not Indicated
FS is generally not indicated when colonoscopy is indicated. It is not indicated for polypectomy because colonoscopy is indicated in these patients, and full colonic preparation is necessary to prevent explosion.

F. Preparation
Two phosphate enemas prior to the examination.

G. Complications
Perforation of the colon occurs in 1 of 10,000 cases.

IV. **Endoscopic Retrograde Cholangiopancreatography (ERCP)**

A. Description
ERCP is a diagnostic procedure for evaluating the pancreatic or biliary tract. It is performed under mild intravenous sedation similar to that used for EGD. The procedure utilizes a lateral-viewing gastroscope placed into the descending duodenum. Upon visualization of the ampulla of Vater, a small plastic catheter is passed through the entire extent of the instrument for entry into the pancreatic or common bile duct. The ductal system is then opacified by injection of iodinated dyes under fluoroscopic monitoring. Radiographs are obtained following contrast injection into the appropriate ductal system. Since most diseases of the pancreas and major biliary ducts present with early ductal abnormalities, the procedure is diagnostically highly accurate.

B. Indications
1. Evaluation of the jaundiced patient suspected of having treatable biliary obstruction.
2. Evaluation of the patient without jaundice whose clinical presentation suggests bile duct disease.

3. Evaluation of signs or symptoms suggesting pancreatic malignancy when results of ultrasound and/or computer tomography are normal or equivocal.
4. Evaluation of recurrent or persistent pancreatitis of unknown etiology.
5. Preoperative evaluation of the patient with chronic pancreatitis.
6. Evaluation of possible pancreatic pseudocyst prior to surgery.
7. Therapeutic endoscopy of the pancreaticobiliary tree, e.g., endoscopic sphincterotomy, balloon dilatation of strictures, and stent placement.

C. Limitations of ERCP
ERCP usually provides no further information when the patient with abdominal pain of obscure origin is subjected to this examination.

D. Preparation for ERCP
Patient should fast for 6 hours prior to the examination. Barium within 48 hours preceding this examination may interfere with radiographic visualization of the common bile duct or pancreatic ducts.

E. Complications
The complication rate is about 2%, with a case-fatality rate of 0.2%. In 1% of cases, acute pancreatitis or recurrence of chronic pancreatitis occurs. In 20–73% of patients, an asymptomatic rise of serum amylase is noted. The possibility of infection is increased when ductal obstruction exists.

V. Antibiotic Prophylaxis for Endoscopy

In patients with prosthetic heart valves or in those who are immunocompromised, neutropenic, or on hemodialysis with a graft fistula, antibiotics are generally indicated for colonoscopy and EGD with biopsy, injection of varices, or dilatation of the esophagus. Ampicillin and gentamicin (one dose) is recommended prior to the endoscopic examination. If penicillin allergy exists, vancomycin should be substituted for ampicillin. Patients with rheumatic valvular heart disease or a past history of endocarditis should probably also have antibiotic prophylaxis. Patients with artificial prostheses such as hip or joint replacements may benefit from similar antibiotic administration. The value of antibiotic prophylaxis in mitral valve prolapse is currently unknown, but if it is prescribed, amoxicillin 3 grams orally may be taken 2 hours prior to the endoscopic examination.

SUGGESTED READING

Sivak MU Jr: *Gastroenterologic Endoscopy*. Philadelphia, WB Saunders, 1987.

Index

Page numbers in *italics* denote figures; those followed by "t" denote tables.